To Sharon
with joy

DON'T FORGET THE COFFEE POT

Dolores Poutré Schwalb

PublishAmerica
Baltimore

First printing

Hardcover 9781462665860
PUBLISHED BY PUBLISHAMERICA, LLLP
www.publishamerica.com
Baltimore

Printed in the United States of America

I would like to dedicate this book to all the people we came to know and love in the delightful little town of New Albany, Pennsylvania. And to my dear husband who took me there. My heart will always be with you. You became, for me, my second "home town" and I thank you.

TABLE OF CONTENTS

CHAPTER 1

Starting Married Life

The sun shone down on us as we walked down the steps of the First Baptist Church in Medford, Oregon. Our car waiting in front was festooned with a paper banner stating; JUST MARRIED in bold happy lettering. Holding the hand of my best friend, now my husband, I smiled up at him as we walked through the hail of rice falling around us, and, I'm sure our hearts were beating as one.

It was May 28, 1950. Mama and Daddy were there smiling their approval. Mama clutched her new purse that matched her shoes, a new dress and hat finished her outfit.

'Mama, take the price tag off your hat, or someone might think your Minnie Pearl. Looking straight at me she quipped;

"What's so bad about that?" But she took it off, just to please me. Daddy had on a suit and tie, and he was standing so stiff he looked like he would break if he bent, his new shoes were shinier than the foil star on our Christmas tree. He was holding a mint toothpick between his fingers in case he got the urged to smoke. If it hadn't been for mama's hat I would have missed all five feet of him. I think he was the smallest adult there. I felt a lump come up in my throat and happy tears threatened to spill out for all the world to see.

My sister, Phyllis, one year older than I, had married a few years back and settled with her farmer husband in Kansas. Barbara, two years behind me married an orchard farmer from Washington state. Tomorrow my husband, Kenneth, and I would leave Oregon, bound for Pennsylvania.

That left only our younger two siblings at home. Janet, six years younger than Barbara and Roger, our baby brother, one year younger than Janet. We were getting scattered clear across America. My sisters often said;

"Dolores, aren't you ever going to get married? You don't even have a boy friend."

It drove them crazy, but I planed to get an education beyond high school and I had only myself to get me there. My parents had just come out of the depression and were still trying to pay off a mortgage on daddy's meager income. They were in no position to help me with further schooling. I had to stay focused and I did get enough education in the arts that I could build on. Then, much to my sisters surprise, along came Kenneth. Our getting acquainted period lasted four years and, well, here we are, me twenty one and Kenneth twenty five, walking through the scattering rice, down the steps of the church on our way to build a life for ourselves. Kenneth looked at me and said,

"Hello, Mrs. Schwalb, are you ready for this?" Grinning, I said;

"I'm never one to turn my back on a challenge." The day before we had closed our bank accounts and would leave for Pennsylvania first thing in the morning. Kenneth's machine shop teacher would be waiting when we got to the little town of New Albany, Pennsylvania. Where there was a small machine shop where Kenneth will finish his training to become a machinist.

Carefully measuring our cash to make it last until we got to Pennsylvania, we planned to camp most of the way and enjoy what our states had preserved for us. Our first night, we would stay at an inexpensive motel on South Riverside in Medford. Kenneth made sure his coffee pot was right up front where he could grab it when we stopped. He told me:

"Coffee gets me going in the morning and fuels me all day." So, the coffee pot was put in a quick to grab position. We left the church amid much whistling, some one called out:

"Good bye, don't forget to write." And we were on our way. Arriving at the motel we ordered a light supper that we ate at our leisure. We wanted to leave early in the morning so we went to bed around nine o'clock.

Kenneth went in to take a shower and get ready for bed, he came out his hair was slicked down like a department store manikins, his pajamas pressed as if he was on display. And the smell was enough to make me swoon. Chuckling to my self I thought;

"Whoo, wee, he sure picked the right after shave." Add a necktie and handkerchief in the pocket you'd think he was advertising for a pajama commercial.

"Boy, I hope he doesn't expect me to be that tidy." Peering out at me from the mirror was an image in a wrinkled nightgown and hair in curlers. Turning out the light I jumped in bed before my slovenly ways could be detected. He didn't say anything, and he never did, all through our marriage he accepted me the way I was.

Tomorrow we would start our journey across the United States from Oregon to Pennsylvania.

The car was packed to overflowing with everything we owned to start our life together. This included three toasters, a waffle iron, and enough bath sets and sheets to last at least eight years. Our suitcases and boxes packed tightly in all the remaining corners. The old coffee pot right on top where it could be reached at a moments notice.

The following morning I woke up to see Kenneth standing in the open door looking out on the world, coffee cup in one hand and the map in the other. He spotted me looking at him,

"Hey, I'm ready when you are, there's a Denney's across the street, we'll catch breakfast there if your ready before lunch." Throwing a pillow at him I remark,

"Oh, yah, I'm faster than lightning when you get me riled." leaping at him like a cat I ran my fingers up his ribs making him almost spill his coffee. Holding me at bay he carefully placed his coffee cup down and chased me around the room his big feet slapping the floor like a giant rabbit.

"This is better." I thought, crumpling in laughter. This day was going to be a camping, sight seeing day so I put on my worn comfortable jeans, a light pullover shirt and my every day tennis shoes, then, I looked at Kenneth in a nice sports coat and slacks, his hair 'party slick. He tossed me a smiled as he walked to the car. The back of his hair looked like it had exploded at the crown pointing in every direction. His coattail caught up in the band of his pants but, what the heck, he thought he looked swell so I didn't say anything. While he was checking to make sure we hadn't forgotten anything I quickly change into some nice slacks, a stylish shirt, and sandals.

"If he wants to go off in style, style it will be." Picking up my suitcase I went out to help him finish packing.

One more look around to check for any forgotten items and to retrieve the little soap samples for hand washing when we stopped at the camp grounds and we were on our way. As he hustled by me, I couldn't resist tweaking his coattail into a more proper alignment. Smiling I stepped out into my new world waiting to be explored. Kenneth got the map out of the glove compartment and made sure everything was neat and orderly inside before he carefully shut the door. Hand in hand, we walked across the street to the restaurant. As we opened the door the breakfast smells rolled out, pancakes, bacon and eggs, with the aroma of coffee holding it all together. The smells turned on the salivary juices and made my stomach tighten. After the light supper we'd had we were more than ready to calm the hunger pangs. A line of people were waiting but, we didn't mind, this was our day and we were in no hurry. We stood quietly watching the people come and go. Every now and then Kenneth squeezed my hand, my heart leaped and I hugged his arm in response. The waitress came to seat us and take our order. While waiting for breakfast, Kenneth laid out the map. He drew a line from Medford to Crater Lake through Klamath Falls and on through the Klamath Indian territory.

"This is the route I took when I came out five years ago." He explained.

"I didn't have much time to stop and enjoy the trip then but, this time, there's no hurry, except to get there before the money runs out and we have to sell our belongings."

"Kenneth, we're not that bad off, and besides, we can always get jobs, were both healthy and not afraid to do a little honest work."

"I know," he said, "just joking." After eating breakfast we climbed back in the 1942 Packard sedan. Smiling broadly, Kenneth gave me a peck on the cheek, the motor came to life and we were off on the ride into our future. My heart lifted with joy. I wanted to hold it forever.

Taking the map I followed our planned route with a pencil but, mostly watched the country roll by. For a person who had only been out of the Rogue Valley only a few times, this was pure excitement. I didn't want to miss a thing as I may never come this way again.

May, what a beautiful month to experience the world around you. The country, just coming awake from the long winter, everything brand new, from the fresh smells of new grass, the gentle greens of the pastures, new foliage on the trees uncurling in anticipation of a new season, blossoms of pink and white and in places along the way some one had planted lilacs.

As we drove Kenneth told me about his relatives that we would meet when we got back East. His aunt and uncle, that he was very fond of in New Jersey, a brother in Poughkeepsie, New York, and cousins in the Bronx. He wanted this to be a total surprise and he was excited at the prospect of arriving unannounced.

"Kenneth, are you sure? They may not be there or they may have other plans. Don't you think you should at least send them a post card letting them know we're coming?" He assured me;

"I know my relatives, they never go anyplace. They didn't think I would ever get married, this will knock them over." Shrugging my shoulders I settled in to enjoying the day. We stopped now and then to take pictures and stretch our legs. Going through the mountains amongst the tall evergreens towering overhead made me feel like an ant. Through my open window floated all the smells of the woodland, the heavy tantalizing smell of the pines and redwoods, an occasional scent of smoke from a camp fire. And the quiet, the heavenly quiet, every sound distinct and isolated from the other. Only the whir of The car's motor like the giant hum of a bee as we cruised along, mile after mile. Arriving at Crater Lake around noon, we pulled into the camp area. Kenneth built a fire and the smell of coffee soon joined the smells of hot dogs, steaks and bacon along with the sizzling sounds of the barbequed meats cooking. After a half-hour break, the coffee pot went back in its place and we were on our way again, traveling through the obsidian mountains, Klamath Indian territory and on to Sprague Park for the night.

The morning of May 30th, our alarm clock woke me at 6:00 a.m. The morning was crisp and cold. So cold, in fact, a basin of water we'd gotten the night before to wash our faces in and freshen up was frozen over. Picking up a rock I broke the ice, taking a deep breath, quickly splashed the cold water on my face, letting out an audible yelp to announce the fact. Kenneth's laugh echoed through the park, but, when I threatened to dump the whole thing down his neck he simmered down a bit. We strolled around the camp to get our circulation going and had a hasty breakfast. Kenneth packed the coffee pot carefully back in its spot. Climbed back in the Packard amongst our belongings, we took off for the second day of our trip. The next stop would be Lakeview. The day went by fast as we whirled along the highway laughing and singing and enjoying our freedom. Arriving at Lakeview we stopped for a few groceries and gassed up. After stretching our legs we were on our way again. Going through lava flow country. An area where there had been a volcanic eruption many years ago. It left the terrain looking like the surface of the moon, or, what I imagined it to look like. By evening we were at Yellowstone and found a campsite in a quiet secluded area at Old Faithful campground. After taking showers we bedded down and were asleep by 10:00 p.m.

May 31st. We got up in time to see Old Faithful erupt. It was a fabulous sight in the early morning. The preliminary bubbling and gurgling with everybody holding their breath for the final swoosh of water shooting high in the morning air. People standing in tight little groups pulled in their breath in an exclamation of awe. After this demonstration of nature at her best we sat a moment on a bench facing the spectacular exhibition to marvel at what we had seen. Little chipmunks came from out of nowhere to beg for nuts or crumbs. We watched them in silent amusement for a while Then, back in the car we drove slowly around the park observing the many animals that were wandering everywhere-moose, deer, bison and several bears One mother bear sent her two cubs scurrying up a tree when we drove by.

Wanting to make good time, we pointed our car in the direction of Rawlins, Wyoming stopping once at a rest stop for a light, quick lunch, then, hurried on our way to our destination, the Seminole rest camp outside of Rawlins, Wyoming. We had covered 333 miles, enough for the day. After a good night's rest, we fixed a quick breakfast and took off for day number four at eight o'clock.

May 32nd—Feeling the grind, we were slower than usual getting started. It was time to find a motel to rest up and do some laundry.

415 miles later, we pulled into a motel in Kearney, Nebraska. It is amazing, I thought how tired I felt and all I did was sit, It was to late to take a walk but, sleeping in a bed that night felt good for a change. The following morning I was up at six and out for a long run to loosen my joints and stir up my blood a bit. Kenneth wasn't a runner like I was but he must have had other ways to deal with the inactivity of his body, however, I never saw him run. But, back home he had taken me skating a few times and he was a whiz on skates. That activity I had watched from the side lines We took our time over breakfast then wandered around town. Kenneth got a pair of work pants and I splurged on a new blouse. After doing the laundry, we went to a favorite local restaurant for a light lunch, then took a long walk. I was refreshed from my morning run and enjoyed the day immensely. We had a full day with the laundry and a little shopping and sight seeing so we stayed at the motel in Kearney a second night. We left early the next morning, June 1st—my enthusiasm had slipped a bit. I was feeling like a soul without roots. I wanted to curl up with a book for a few hours and be alone. I felt guilty for even thinking this, but I noticed that Kenneth was spending a lot of time gazing off across the countryside in a sort of trance. His mind was somewhere else. I think we both felt saturated, like two kids who had been too long at the fair.

We had never been together this long at one stretch and needed time to sort through our feelings. We would overcome this in time.

That night we camped at Lake of Three Fires in Belford, Iowa. It stormed during the night with a lot of thunder and lightning. It was still storming in the morning and we hurriedly ate breakfast and got on our way, hoping to get out of the storm. We drove through a small town where the streets were littered with leaves, and branches, cars looked like they had been beaten with a ball peen hammer, and there were hail stones on the ground the size of golf balls. The storm had left a mess for the folks here to clean up.

When we stopped outside of town for a light lunch, I couldn't find the coffee pot. It was not on its perch. I realized that I had forgotten to put it back in the car and it was still sitting at our campsite in Belford. Kenneth was very unhappy. He looked daggers at me and said, "I can't believe you left the coffee pot, of all things." He was quiet and grumpy all morning. I felt miserable. We stopped at a small town and got another pot. I vowed that I would not forget this one; it would be my primary responsibility.

That night, we stayed at a camp ground in Peru, Illinois. The following morning, we counted our cash and decided not to tarry. We were running low on funds and had about enough money left to get us to Dick Byrons with one more stop at a motel. Driving steadily on through Indiana and Ohio, late that evening, we pulled across the line into Pennsylvania.

CHAPTER 2

We Arrive in Pennsylvania

Something looked strange. I couldn't decide what it was but something was very different. Gazing at the landscape going by, it dawned on me. It was the telephone poles. They were knobby, like crooked trees with their branches trimmed. It made me feel like we were driving through the "crooked man" territory, like the poem, "There was a crooked man, that walked a crooked mile." Coming from Oregon where you take straight telephone poles for granted, they looked weird to me: it made the passing landscape look like a cartoon strip. I didn't see any tall pine trees growing on the hills; in fact, there were no straight trees anywhere.

We passed immaculately-kept farms with barns decorated with Hex signs. A herd of milk cows were grazing in the fields, some walking in long lines heading toward the barns.

"It must be milking time," Kenneth said.

"I know, but I sure wouldn't want to milk that many cows all in one evening."

Kenneth laughed, and told me, "They are milked by machine."

"That must be very uncomfortable for the cows, no soft warm hands to pull their teats and pat their sides or talk to them, how sad." He grinned and said, "They're used to being milked that way and the machines are very gentle." I still thought the farmer and the cow were missing something very special.

We finally arrived in the little town of Towanda, Pennsylvania. There were no motels but we found a bed and breakfast. The proprietors fixed us a light supper and after taking showers, we went to bed. The next morning we were up early, anxious to be on our way.

After breakfast, Kenneth showed me around Towanda. This was the town where we would do most of our shopping. There was one main street going straight through town with two parallel streets on either side, connected by three or four side streets. You could stand in the middle of town and see both ends clearly. I thought Medford was small but Towanda had Medford beat. If you blinked, you would miss the whole town. I spotted a bank, drugstore, Sears catalogue store, and two or three clothing stores.

As we were leaving town, we passed the Mills hospital. A couple of blocks beyond the hospital was a secondhand store that would become my favorite place to shop. We drove past the tiny town of Monroton, and then followed the winding roads flanked on both sides by dense wooded hills, where we saw only a couple of ramshackle houses tucked back in the trees.

After driving about ten or twelve miles we arrived at New Albany, Pennsylvania. It was a neat orderly little town with two churches, the First Baptist and the Methodist, a gas station and mortuary combined, Bouse's hardware, a large feed mill, two small grocery stores, bank, post office and a large wreath factory that took up two blocks. On the edge of town was a restaurant, another one in the middle of town, and next to the post office was the Shady Nook, a small coffee shop where the town people gathered for morning coffee and gossip. I had not seen any saloons anywhere. I learned later that this was a completely "dry" town, no liquor allowed.

Following a road out of town that veered to the right, we finally found the little town of Overton where Dick's cousins, Agnes and Mary Ellen Leigh, lived.

The only buildings in Overton were a Catholic church, a post office and a large rambling two-story house that stood beyond the church.

Kenneth drove up to the house and two women came out. One was skinny and as flighty as a chicken just let out of her coop. The other one was slow and plump—like a big balloon, she floated. Both were gray-haired and dressed in cotton dresses made from floral printed feed sacks. Agnes and Mary Ellen Leigh were sisters, Irish from the soles of their farm shoes to the top of their gray flyaway buns. With their little aprons aflutter, they invited us in. We chatted a few minutes, and then they told us how to get to Dick and Jessie's place just a few miles up the road. We thanked them and headed for Dick's. When we arrived, they were expecting us and greeted us with open arms. I felt instantly at home. I liked these people and would grow fond of them over the next few years.

Jessie was walking with a cane. She had recently had hip surgery and was still on the mend, but in spite of that, her movements were quick and efficient. You could tell that she was an "in charge" person. There was a professional aura about her. I learned later that she had been a head nurse at a hospital in New York City before she retired.

They had a beautiful well-groomed collie dog that they called Mazy. She stood up, wagged her tail in greeting, then lay down on a blanket by Dick's chair.

The house took me back to my childhood, a typical farmhouse with no running water, but a pitcher pump in the kitchen, marble-topped counters, and cupboards galore. The ceilings were at least eight feet high. The floors were wide-planked boards with braided cotton throw rugs in strategic spots. A large black and chrome cooking stove, with a warming oven over the top, was the focal point of the country kitchen. Out the back door down the path from the house was the outdoor privy.

The house smelled of fresh air and floor polish. She showed us to the guest room and after we took our suitcases in she offered us glasses of ice tea, a real treat after our long trek. Dick was a short, round-shouldered man. He looked uncomfortable in stiff new farm clothes but he was trying to put on the look of a farmer. From all the years he had sat behind a desk. Trying to make the transition from a city dweller to a farmer took some practice. He kept reaching to adjust his tie, which was no longer there.

We chatted about our plans. Kenneth asked Dick where he thought he might get a job in a hurry. Dick told him he could get a job on the road breaking rock: they were always shorthanded. He offered to take him there Monday. This was Friday, so we had a couple of days to get acquainted with the territory. We were so tired that we just wanted a little time to relax. Getting used to the basin and outhouse again was a drag. The following morning, I awoke early to take my sojourn down the well-worn path. I had gotten a nice salmon-colored satin bathrobe. It felt good to put on nice things after a week in jeans and tennis shoes. I put on my robe and stood a minute hugging up the luxury of the fabric, then headed for the outhouse. As I went through the kitchen I greeted Jessie getting breakfast.

She said, "Good morning," then took one horrified look at me and called Kenneth. He came running out, looking like he was part porcupine with his hair in all directions, his eyes wide open, and startled.

"What's wrong?"

"You can't let her go out in that beautiful robe: you'll have to carry her." Jessie said. He looked at me in disbelief and I looked back at him. No way was I going to let him carry me: I wanted to get there in one piece.

"It's okay, Jessie," I said, "I'll hold the robe up so it won't get soiled," and I made a hasty dash for the door.

That afternoon, we went on a hike up in the hills around the fence line of Dick's property. It was dense with trees, lots of maples, sumac and oak. The weekend went by fast. By Monday, it had been decided that we would stay with Agnes and Mary Ellen because they could use our services to fix fences and take care of their animals—a few cows and chickens. They had a lot of repair work to do and we felt good that we could make ourselves useful.

Kenneth started his road job early Monday morning: Jessie packed him a lunch and off he went.

That afternoon, Dick hooked up a team of horses to a plow. It was a little more sophisticated than the one Daddy used: this one had a seat on it. You could sit on it holding the reins to guide the horses. It looked like fun. I asked Dick if I could try it.

"Okay, just don't let the horses go too fast." he cautioned. "Pull back on the reins and they'll slow down." I was having a blast when Jessie came hobbling out, waving her cane wildly over her head and yelling.

"Dick! Dick! What are you doing? She could kill herself. Then what would Kenneth say?" She was in a frenzy. I had to convince her that I was pretty hardy and didn't break easily. She would get used to me in time.

Kenneth arrived a little after five. I went out to greet him and find out how his day had gone. He put one foot out of the car and then the other one. His bright white socks were not bright white anymore: they were both blood-red down to his shoes. I stopped and looked in horror at my poor husband.

"My gosh, what happened?" I asked.

"Well, I didn't know there was a right and wrong way to hit a rock," he quipped, "but I do now. You're supposed to hit it so it flies away from your shins not into them. I'm learning." His poor shins looked like someone had used them for target practice and were pretty good at hitting their target. I got him bandaged up and soaked his socks in a little Clorox water, my first performance as a good wife. I was in business.

CHAPTER 3

Life on the Leigh Farm

The next day, we moved in with Agnes and Mary Ellen. They had a huge two-story house and took in hunters during hunting season. We were given a nice big room at the head of the stairs with a small private porch and entrance at the bottom.

Their dining room was big enough to skate in. The table had a big bouquet of roses in the center and at each end were large spoon holders and a set of salt and pepper shakers. The table was so long you felt like you had to pass notes from one end to the other to communicate. The ladies showed us around the farm, pointing out things we could do to spruce the place up.

Agnes had been married and it was her husband who had built the house. He had been repairing the roof when he fell and lost his life. Everything was just as he had left it, including an old rusty Ford in the garage. It was new at the time of his accident, but time had taken its toll and it now housed big black spiders. For as long as we were there, no one went near it.

That evening, after a wonderful supper, we both took luxurious baths and sank into a very comfortable bed. Ah! Sweet bliss. The following morning, we were up early—Kenneth to go to his rock breaking job and I to learn about life on the Leigh farm.

I went down to greet the sisters. I wanted to whistle or sing to let the world know how great I felt.

Mary Ellen had a bucket of "rocks she was pouring in the stove (At this point, I should remind you that I'm from the little Rogue Valley in Oregon where we never see coal; I learned about it in school but never had an opportunity to observe it in use.) She looked up and said; "Good morning." and kept right on with her pouring.

"Mary Ellen, what are you doing?" I asked. I suppose I sounded a little anxious and she looked at me in alarm.

"Building a fire."

"With rocks?"

She threw back her head and laughed. Then wiping her eyes, she explained to me that this was coal. Another lesson learned. Coal may look like rocks, but it's <u>not</u>!

Some of the terms these two ladies used had a definite Irish twist. Mary Ellen was the doer of the two and did most of the active work, so I stuck with her and tried to learn her routine. After she showed me how to put coal on the fire, we started outside with a bag of trash.

"Where are we going now?" I asked.

Looking at me over her shoulder, she answered, "To the thrash."

I repeated, "The thrash?"

"Yes, you know the 'gargage'." I translated that to mean, garbage. I thought I was getting pretty smart—"thrash" was trash and "gargage" was garbage. This was going to be a fun learning experience. That weekend, Dick told Kenneth he had a field of buckwheat that the deer were raiding and he would love it if he could down one or two of them. The farmers had permission to hunt the deer out of season if they were ruining their crops. Kenneth was very happy to oblige.

Saturday evening about dusk, he told me we were going to help Dick save his buckwheat crop from the raiding deer and he wanted me to come along to hold the flashlight. He took his rifle and headed for the field. I followed along to learn another survival trick. I felt like a real pioneer. We waited at the edge of the field, quietly, watching, until the silhouette of a deer appeared. Kenneth whispered;

"Turn your flashlight on it." I turned the beam in the direction of the silhouette, at the same time Kenneth pulled the trigger. There was a resounding boom! Jumping backward, I stumbled on a root and fell with a thud on my derrière. The sound of the shot plus my earth shaking crash must have cleared the whole mountain of any small critters that had plans of spending the night. But, the deed was done. When we got across the field, there lay our winter's meat with its tongue hanging out. Kenneth managed to drag the deer to the edge of the field and after taking out the innards, it became lighter. He lifted it on Dick's tractor and drove it to Agnes's barn to hang until it "cooled out." This was all new to me, but I was learning.

The following day, Kenneth took the deer carcass down and moved it into the laundry room where Agnes and Mary Ellen took over. They packaged, labeled and stored it in their freezer. Two days later, I went to the laundry room to wash some clothes and just about lost my breakfast on the spot. They had not cleaned up the mess from the deer cutting and there were a million little wiggly maggots trying to do the job for them. I couldn't handle it. I flew out of there in a hurry, gagging and choking as I went. When Kenneth came home, I was in our room having a big crying jag.

"What's wrong?" he asked. I couldn't tell him, so I took him to the laundry room and let him see for himself. I stood there gagging, with tears streaming down my face. He got a couple of buckets of very hot water and started flushing the place out. In about half an hour, it was as clean as a baby's nursery. I felt like I had failed as a housewife and told him how sorry I was.

Forget it," he said, patting me on the back. "You'll get used to this sort of thing in time." I vowed that I never would, and right then and there became a fanatic about keeping things clean.

Kenneth and I spent many hours fixing fences and generally sprucing up the place. This would compensate for our room and board, but we needed some means of income. Kenneth's rock breaking job was not enough.

Agnes had a good idea. She offered to advance us enough money to get 50 baby chicks. We could raise and sell them at broiler stage. There was an empty chicken coop in the backyard that we could use and they would teach me the ins and outs of raising chickens. I knew chickens but ours back home more or less took care of themselves. This would be a bit different.

That weekend, we got the chicks and put them in the coop under a brooder. The light had to be kept on so they wouldn't stack up and smother themselves. When they were a week old, I let them out of the coop during the day and kept their water containers and feed troughs filled. At dusk, I turned on the lights in the coop and they would all go in for the night. Mary Ellen told me not to forget to turn the lights on at the proper time or they would pile up and suffocate. It was a chicken's natural tendency to climb to a high level to roost, and if they couldn't see, they would climb on top of one another and smother. I took very good care of my chickens and they grew nicely. They were almost big enough for market. Then one evening, I forgot to turn the lights on. When I realized the sun had gone down, I dashed out to the coop. My chickens were stacked in a big feathery heap up against the door. There was no movement from them. I called franticly for help. Agnes and Mary Ellen came rushing out of the house. As I stood looking on in horror, Mary Ellen started grabbing the chickens by the neck, whirling them in the air. Agnes grabbed an ax, chopped off their heads and hung them on the clothes line. In just a short time, 50 headless chickens were hanging on the line by their feet. Mary Ellen brought out a big tub and filled it with hot water. She told to me to grab a chicken, dip it in hot water and pull off the feathers. They were moving so fast I was caught up in the urgency of what had to be done. I did what they told me and was grabbing chickens and ripping feathers like a person possessed. It was like trying to catch a runaway train. They didn't even give me time to mourn the loss of my charges.

The next step was gutting them. The two sisters showed me how to pull the entrails out, find the heart, gizzard, and liver and separate them from the other entrails and drop them in a pan of ice water. Agnes grabbed each chicken after it was cleaned and dipped it first in very hot water then in ice water. She explained that this plumped them and made them look good to the grocer. By two o'clock in the morning fifty chickens were ready for market. I was too tired to have any feelings about the matter. All I wanted was to go to bed and sleep for a week.

The following day, Kenneth took the chickens into New Albany and sold them to the local grocer. We paid Agnes and had a little left over for ourselves. I had gained a new skill-how to clean a chicken in a hurry.

Wednesday of the following week, Agnes and Mary Ellen had to go to town and invited me to come along. Apparently, this was something they did on very rare occasions and they made a big to-do about it. They both came down dressed in their best. Agnes's adopted daughter, Ann, came to pick us up. When she arrived, Agnes got in the front seat with Ann and Mary Ellen started to climb in the back. I looked at her and she had a big black smudge on her forehead. I told her about it.

"That's okay," she said, "This is Ash Wednesday." She got in the back seat of the car. Then I noticed they all had the same smudge on their foreheads. (I had learned one thing and that is, if you don't know what's going on, keep your mouth shut. I did just that. I would pick up clues along the way.) I later came to understand that it had something to do with their religion. I didn't know much about the Catholic faith but I would find out a lot from these ladies.

I still needed to get a job, and knowing there was a wreath factory in town, I thought I would try there. Having made wreaths at Harry and David's fruit packing plant in Medford, I felt it would be a snap. I was wrong. I was told that they only hired people who had experience in making wreaths their way. I didn't qualify.

One evening, two of Agnes and Mary Ellen's young nephews brought over several bags of Princes Pine, which was what the factory used for making the wreaths. The boys were going to teach me how to make wreaths the way the factory wanted them made, and then I could apply for work as a trained wreath maker.

They got a big washtub and filled it with water then dumped a bag of the Princes Pine in it. After it had soaked for an hour, they brought out some small rolls of wire and taught me the fine art of wreath making. I practiced until I had used up all the pine they had brought. When

Monday morning came, I was ready. The boys took me to the wreath factory in New Albany and I applied for a job. They told me to come in the next day to start work. My starting wage would be 75 cents an hour. There was joy in my soul.

When Kenneth came home that evening, I told him the good news and he hugged Me, nearly knocking me off my feet and said,

"Now it's my turn to give you my good news. We are moving into our own house in New Albany this weekend. Mr. Slocum has a house that he will rent to us for only 25 dollars a month and I will start work Monday at the machine shop just a few blocks from where we will live." His starting wage would be $ 1.50 per hour. Hurray! We're on our way!

CHAPTER 4

Our First Home

We had not unpacked our boxed belongings since we left Medford because we were waiting for this moment when we could unpack them and put things on shelves or in drawers. Kenneth had told me not to get dishes for eating, as he had plenty that he'd brought with him from New York and they were still packed. It would be like Christmas in July.

Saturday, we drove to Towanda and purchased our first piece of furniture, a hide-a-bed. It would serve as a bed at night and as a couch during the day. They delivered it that same afternoon and I unpacked our brand-new bedding and a couch throw.

In the dinning room were a large table and eight chairs. There was no need to purchase any more furniture at this time. We would make do and get items one at a time as the need arose.

Kenneth got his little foldaway camp stove, one of the toasters, the waffle iron and of course, the coffee pot, and put them in the kitchen. We made it through that first week using what we had. I even made a sponge cake using my waffle iron, putting wild strawberries and whipped cream between the layers, it made a luscious desert. Kenneth thought I was great! He didn't know the worst of me yet, but he would soon find out. I had never cooked anything but pork roast, which I hated, and I had made a few salads, at Mama's request but, my culinary skills were pretty meager.

We opened the boxes of pots and pans that Kenneth had gotten me as a wedding gift—a complete set of Revere Ware stainless steel with a life time guarantee. After fifty seven years, I still have every piece, even the small saucepan that survived being used as a hammer. Any time I needed a hammer and didn't want to go to Kenneth's tool chest, I would use the little saucepan. It had a solid bottom and a sturdy handle and it was always available. (it was repaired three times.) The large chicken fryer lost its handle from heavy use over the years, but with no handle, it was perfect for making Dutch Baby pancakes that had to be made in the oven. But now, they were brand new. The copper bottoms were so beautiful I had Kenneth make a rack so I could hang them on the wall. The pans added a touch of elegance to my kitchen.

We had been married almost two months and now lived in our first rented home, had jobs, a bed and couch combination, and all the kettles we would ever need for the rest of our lives. Living one block from the local hardware store made it handy to purchase needed items as our cash flow strengthened. The first items were a clothes basket and clothes pins. I have numerous items that I still use that came from Bouse's hardware store.

After getting everything arranged in the house, Kenneth brought in two large boxes that he had carefully packed. Opening them he started pulling out cups, saucers, plates, etc, all museum quality china. Nothing matched, the pieces were all signed and dated by his grandfather. I was shocked! I could never use these dishes: they were family treasures to be cherished. There were tiny demitasse cups and saucers, delicate individual soup tureens, plates with photos of Kenneth's mother and father etched into them, several sample plates with family crests numbered around the edge. Kenneth explained to me that if a piece of china was broken, the owner only had to point out his pattern and order the proper piece to be replaced from these sample plates. In one of the boxes there was a small ledger with some of the formulas for different techniques in china decorating.

In the early 1900s, Kenneth's grandfather operated a china factory where he designed and decorated china for the big families of New York. The dishes that Kenneth had inherited were the sample pieces that had been displayed in his shop. We packed them carefully away and went to Grants to get an inexpensive but nice set of Melmac.

CHAPTER 5

Meeting Kenneth's Relatives

The following weekend, we took some time off and went to New York to pay Kenneth's relatives a surprise visit. I was apprehensive about popping in on people and thought we should call ahead and let them know we were coming. Kenneth still insisted that he wanted to surprise them, so off we went, unannounced, to meet the relatives. When we arrived in New York, we drove to the Bronx and checked into a hotel Near where Kenneth's cousins lived The following morning, we went to their apartment. It was in a very tall depressing gray building. The old elevator creaked and complained the three floors up. When it came to a rattling halt, we stepped off into a poorly lit hall, heavy with the smell of stale cigarette smoke and cooking odors. Kenneth walked right to their door. He said they had lived there for years and he knew the place by heart. After ringing the bell, we waited for a short minute. A frizzle-haired, anxious-looking woman opened the door. When she saw Kenneth, she let out a shrill nasal scream that should have awakened everybody in the whole building. This was his cousin's wife. Yelling for her husband to come quickly she nearly smothered Kenneth in a bear hug. Pounding him on the back, she repeated over and over in her high nasal pitch,

It's Kenneth! It's Kenneth!" She gathered her apron up, wrapping her arms in it and asked us to, "Come on in, I thought you were still out west, my, my what a surprise." Her husband came ambling out of somewhere, clutching a newspaper, wearing no shirt. Baggy pants supported by wide red suspenders: and a pair of shabby run-over slippers were on his feet. His hair was sticking up like a porcupine. I thought this kind of hair must run in the family: it was just like Kenneth's before it was combed. The air was filled with excitement, everyone laughing and talking at once. I had heard that people in the Bronx have a distinctly different way of talking and this was it—I hardly understood a word they were saying. Two pale-looking children, a boy about ten and a girl around eight, came quietly out of the background. The girl, who seemed to be the youngest, peeked around her brother, a bedraggled rag doll in one hand. The boy, wearing faded overalls, his little bony arms hanging limply at his side, stood looking at the goings on. Their dad said,

"Remember the kids? They've grown some since you saw them last." He took them by their shoulders and shoved them into the foreground as if he were showing off his trophies.

"Say hello to Kenneth, kids."

They both said a dull "Hullo," then scooted into the background again. Kenneth's cousin was a fireman, (that explained the suspenders). He worked long hours and had only one week off a year. They spent most of that time hanging around their apartment watching television. The children had never been to a park or seen a tree. We visited for a while over a cup of tea and some store-bought cookies. The wife kept saying in her shrill nasal twang.

"You should have let us know you were coming, I could have baked something." Kenneth said he had wanted to surprise everyone. His cousin said;

"Well, you sure did that, alright, we would have never guessed." The wife went to the kitchen to get more tea and I heard the little girl talking to her, "That lady with Kenneth talks like a foreigner, Mama." Her mother told her. "She is, honey. She's from the West, way out in Oregon." Kenneth told me later that the children had never been out of the Bronx. We visited for about an hour, Kenneth filling them in on the happenings of the past few years and of his sister, Venita, having phlebitis after her baby was born. He had gone to Oregon to help her, where, he explained, he met me. His cousin kept repeating,

"Small world," and "Ya' never know." Kenneth told them that we were going to see another one of the cousins and they said

"Are you sure ya' wanna do that?" Kenneth told them yes: he wanted me to meet the whole family, good and bad. We said our goodbyes and left.

When we got to the street, I looked up and the two children were leaning out of the window three floors up. If I were the mother, I would have been terrified. It was a long way down. Our next visit was in the same area, a little nicer establishment in a taller building. The elevator was quieter, the halls wider and well lit, smelling of disinfectant. These would be more of Kenneth's cousins. When we got to their floor, Kenneth looked at me with a grim determined look on his face. He straightened his tie and squared his shoulders before he rang the doorbell. We heard a muffled sound like a chair moving and some quiet talking before the door opened. Another cousin stood before him and stared at him like he'd expected a peddler and was ready to tell him that he wasn't interested in what he had to offer. He said

"Where did you come from? We're having a birthday party here."

"I just dropped by to introduce you to my wife. We've come a long way and I want her to meet my relatives." Kenneth said.

"You may as well come on in." his cousin said. What a cold atmosphere. These cousins weren't anything like the other family. Why in the world were we here? If I had known what they were like, I never would have set foot in the place. I wanted to get this over with and get out of there. I stepped dutifully inside and was introduced to the cousins. I wished the birthday person a happy birthday and apologized for interrupting their party. Grabbing Kenneth's coattail, I gave it a meaningful tug, pulling him toward the door. Kenneth was humiliated and turned to his cousin and said,

"Nice impression you made on my wife." We turned and left. Kenneth was so upset he was grumpy.

"Hey! Don't be so mad I said, you didn't do anything wrong. They're the ones who humiliated themselves. Every family has some of those kinds but most try to keep them out of sight for their own good. No more surprises, okay?" I never saw them again. We went back to the hotel and Kenneth decided that he would call his aunt and uncle before he went to New Jersey to visit them and make sure we were welcome before going the distance. His aunt was very excited. She said that she would be working the following day but asked Kenneth to come for supper and spend the evening with them. His Uncle Walter was Kenneth's father's only brother. He worked as a broker on Wall Street. Aunt Dorothy had a chain of dress shops throughout New Jersey called the Dorothy Carol dress shops. She and her sisters had started a lingerie factory after their parents died, leaving the four young girls without support. They had opened the dress shops one at a time, as the business grew. The following day, Kenneth took me to his aunt and uncle's home in the suburbs of Ho Ho-Kus, New Jersey. They were wonderful, warm, friendly people. Aunt Dorothy had prepared a delicious German supper of Rolardin, potato dumplings and a tasty salad. She used her nice milk glass dishes and served everyone herself. Placing the food on the plates, she passed them around until everyone was served. I received my plate first and sat waiting for everyone else. I heard a loud pop and to my horror, my plate split in half. Poor Dorothy was distraught.

"Quick, move your food around on your plates the food is too hot for them." She Apologized, saying,

"The plates were too cold; I should have taken them out of the cupboard and let them get to room temperature." They were her mother's milk glass dishes that she had inherited. I felt very sad for her. In spite of the dish breaking, we had a wonderful visit, and when we left, Aunt Dorothy hugged me and said she hoped that we would come often. They made me feel like family. When we got back home, we prepared ourselves for the approaching holidays, my first season away from home. I was determined to make it as festive as I could. Kenneth's boss gave him a 25-pound turkey for Thanksgiving. Jessie loaned me a large electric roaster to cook it in. It barely fit, but we managed to get it cooked. To consume it was another thing. We didn't have a refrigerator yet, so Kenneth buried the pan, with the turkey in it, in the snow to keep it cold. I imagined the pilgrims having to do something like that. We ate turkey until we couldn't stand the looks of it anymore, then put it out in pans for the neighborhood dogs. Winter had come and I was excited to wake up and see the whole town looking like a winter wonderland. Icicles hung like small baseball bats from the eaves. I went outside and my two feet promptly went skyward; I ended up seeing stars in broad daylight. My way of walking to the post office several blocks away must have given the neighbors something to talk about. As I went by the houses holding tightly onto two sticks to keep myself upright, I would see the curtains moving, one house after another, all the way to the post office. I finally got over my fear of falling and got quite good at keeping my balance. With the first paycheck in December, We decided we could afford a used cook stove. The house was heated by a little "bucket a day" coal-burning furnace, and was quite comfortable. We put a bucket of coal in it every morning and it kept us cozy all day. At night, before we went to bed, we put in another bucket and it was cozy all night, but, we were still using our camp stove and waffle iron for cooking. It was time to get a stove. Kenneth borrowed a friend's truck and headed for Dushore to the secondhand store on his quest for a stove. I walked to the feed store about two blocks away and got some green-and-white checked feed sacks to make curtains for the kitchen. About an hour later, Kenneth was back with the stove. It was white and chrome with a big warming oven over the top and a water reservoir to the side. It looked great. I planned on baking a cake as soon as I could, maybe tomorrow for Sunday dinner. After we got it unload and set up I polished it down with my cleaning rag just to give it my, welcome pat and Kenneth went to the coal yard off the ally behind us to get some coal. we were all set to start a fire when the doorbell rang. The house had one of those old doorbells that you had to crank and it started ringing like crazy. It had such an insistent buzzing ring that it raised the hairs on your neck. Kenneth rushed to answer it. When he came back, he didn't look too happy. He said,

"Don't build a fire yet; we have to take the stove back."

"What, that can't be. We just got it and it's paid for, so what's the deal?" A young couple going through a divorce had brought all their furniture to the secondhand store to sell, but had changed their minds, and now wanted all their furniture back. The store owner assured Kenneth that he had another stove he could have at the same price. So back went my nice white stove and a shocking bright blue stove with generous amounts of chrome arrived. I had never seen a blue stove before. There went my vision of a sparkling white kitchen with touches of green. This was going to be our stove for the next five years, like it or not. I took the green-checked feed sacks back and got plain white. I wasn't taking any chances on more changes. I would stick with white for as long as we were still renting. The next day, I baked a German chocolate cake. Ken was proud of me, so he decided to return the favor by planning a surprise. He got a sly grin on his face and said,

"I'm going to the store. I'll be right back." When he returned, I watched him as he came in the back door with a couple of bottles behind his back. The bottles were shaped like beer bottles. It can't be—he would never do that to me. I sat on the couch in frozen shock.

"What's going on?" I thought. "Do I really know this guy?" He called out,

"Don't peek." It was too late for that. I sat there like a stone, shrinking inside myself. He went outside and broke the tips off several icicles hanging off the eaves and stuck them in two glasses, then went back in the kitchen. I heard something pouring into the glasses and he came walking proudly in and handed me a glass. I looked at him stonily and said,

"What is that? I saw you and I know it's beer." He looked crushed. He went back in the kitchen and brought out an empty bottle. It said, "Dad's Old Fashioned Root Beer" on the side. Small, mean and miserable, were good descriptive words for me at that moment. How could I think he would do such a thing to me? I couldn't apologize enough.

He kept saying, "That's okay. Just forget it."

That afternoon, he gathered up some pop bottles and took them to the store to redeem them. When he came back, he had two bags of popcorn. He stood there with his famous smirk and said,

"Want to go to a movie? The guy at the store gave me two bags of popcorn, we can't waste them." We went to a movie for the first time since we had left Medford.

Christmas was just a week away. This would be the first time I had ever been away from home on Christmas. I was trying to stay occupied and keep my mind busy. We had started going to the Evergreen Christian Church a few miles out of New Albany, mainly because we had met some of the young married couples who went there. It was a friendly church and they made us feel at home. They had a choir and the music was warming to the soul. The children put on a very touching Christmas play. It was a real Currier and Ives Christmas. I thanked God for bringing us to this wonderful little community.

At home, I created a huge decoration for the dining room table and we got a small Christmas tree, trimming it with handmade ornaments and popcorn. A large paper angel went on top. Paper snowflakes dotted the windows and, all in all, it looked like Christmas.

We had decided to splurge on the makings of a nice Christmas dinner. I got ham, Brussels sprouts, yams, and made my auntie's famous Waldorf salad. Later in the afternoon we had gingerbread cake and ice cream. I went to the kitchen to make Kenneth some coffee and our funny doorbell rang. When I went to answer it there was no one there, but sitting on the porch beside the door was a big plate of homemade cookies. The donor had fled. I picked them up and smiled at whoever might be watching and took them in the house to share with Kenneth.

I missed my family but I made it through the holidays by just staying focused on the activities going on around town. New Years Day came and we fixed another small dinner and went to a movie. A few days into January, I woke up one morning feeling blah. I didn't think much of it, but the following morning I felt the same way. I had the blahs for a whole week before it dawned on me what my problem was: I was pregnant! Oh! My! Gosh! We're going to have a baby. I made an appointment with Doctor Baker in Towanda at the suggestion of my new friends. He confirmed the fact that, yes indeed, I was with child. Kenneth looked absolutely stunned. The doctor told me what to watch for and how to take care of my health. Kenneth got a whole case of oranges. I never knew what that was all about, but I guess he thought oranges would keep me healthy. We had to throw some of them away—there were too many and they started to spoil.

With Kenneth working at the machine shop, his clothes got very dirty and oily. I had no washing machine and had to wash the clothes in the bathtub. I put special detergents in, then enough water to cover the clothes, climbed in and stomped up and down until I felt they were clean; then I drained the water out and added the rinse water, and stomped them until all the soap was gone and the water was clear. It was quite a chore but he always had nice clean clothes. It sure did wonders for my feet, no "ring around the ankles" on me. Since the maggot incident I had become a clean freak. Kenneth told me that he worried about me having to do laundry like this, and we should start saving for a washing machine. That sounded great. With a baby on the horizon, we would definitely need one. My mother always took care of babies while I was growing up and I was aware of what I was getting into. So, we started a washing machine fund.

The following week Kenneth got a letter from his sister, Venita, in Medford, Oregon. Her husband, Walter, was going back into the Marine Corps and would be stationed in Quantico, Virginia. They would be leaving Medford in a few weeks. Their little girl, Susie, was two years old now and they asked if we could take her for the week that they would be getting settled in Quantico. I was delighted; this would give me an opportunity to have some hands-on experience with a small child before my upcoming challenge.

The weather was still nice when they arrived, so we had a chance to show them around town. Thank goodness they didn't stay overnight because we had no place to put them, we got the mattress from our 'camper' and put it on the floor for Susie. I had a wonderful week showing off Kenneth's niece then, it was time to take her to her mama and daddy.

Traveling with a small child in the backseat had its drawbacks, however. She was restless and didn't want to lie down and sleep, as I had hoped she would. We stopped and I gave her a light lunch, then continued on our way. About a half-hour later her lunch reappeared all over our backseat. Kenneth was frantic-his beloved car that he took such good care of was ruined! We stopped at a house and asked if we could get some water to clean up the mess. A woman answered the door. When Kenneth explained what had happened, she became all authority. She said, "I have several children and this has happened to me more than once." Going in the house she soon reappeared with her cleaning paraphernalia and had the mess cleaned up in minutes. She gave me a pill that she said she used for her children for car sickness. I gave it to Susie. We thanked her profusely and got her name and address. When we got back I sent her a box of candy as a thank you gift. One more lesson learned that day; How to clean a car when a child gets carsick. All these little 'lessons I was picking up along the way would become very helpful in the next few years.

During the summer, I met more of the young married women in town. They had all lived there all of their lives, pretty much like I had lived in Medford, Oregon. They married their high school sweethearts and settled in the same town they grew up in. Most of their husbands were farmers but some worked for the railroad or the factories in nearby towns.

We got an invitation to their high school alumni banquet held in the Fire Hall on a Saturday evening and had a wonderful time getting to know our new neighbors. They planned to put on a play the following month and asked if anyone would take on the task of painting a backdrop for it. My ears perked up and I thought.

"Here is a way I can show my appreciation for their kindness and generosity." I told them that I would be glad to do it for them, as I had a little art training. Some of them didn't think they should involve a stranger, but I convinced them I just wanted to return their friendship and they gave me the job. I felt useful and as if I belonged for the first time since I left home. The men built the framework for the backdrop and covered it with cardboard. The theme was a country Western musical. I painted the outside of a log cabin with an old dented washtub hanging on the side. As an extra, I put a large stump in front of the backdrop and buried an axe in it. I arranged a few well-used barrels to sit on toward the front of the stage. It turned out great and they all liked it, even the skeptics.

Kenneth and I got an invitation to see the performance and I thought, for a small town, they had some real talent. It was fun. We were getting to be known in town as the "newcomers" and got invited to a lot of the town get-togethers.

At the same time, we were collecting more and more necessary items for our coming event. A clothes basket and clothes pins, a bassinet, and most importantly, a washing machine. It was a Maytag with an automatic pump to pump the water out when the washing was finished.

January and February went by pretty smoothly. Then I began to swell up like a puff adder. My dress sleeves got tight and my ankles looked like stuffed sausages. The doctor said that I had edema and had to refrain from using salt. That seemed to help and my puffiness subsided, but my food was bland and not interesting, and I began to lose weight. The doctor didn't like that either and gave me some tips on how to liven up my meals by substituting different spices to take the place of salt. I finally came to grips with it, and to this day. I do not use salt. Even Kenneth got used to my new way of eating.

CHAPTER 6

Our Second Move
The House on the Hill

Our landlord had a relative who was getting married and they wanted the house for him. They told us we would have to move.

Kenneth asked around and we found a place a few miles out of New Albany in Evergreen. The tiny town had a church, grocery store and Irene's Photographers Studio. The house was owned by a dairy farmer. It was on a hill across the road from their barn. A nice wide porch extended completely across the front and opened into the kitchen on one end. A living room was on the other. Stairs went to the upper floor between the kitchen and the living room.

Kenneth borrowed a pickup from one of the workers at the machine shop and we moved the following Saturday. We still didn't have much, but the hide-a-bed and washing machine necessitated the need for the pickup. His friend said that he had a small refrigerator that we could have for $25.00 Kenneth thought that was a good deal so he bought it, loaded it on the truck, and brought it along. It was an ancient G.E. refrigerator with the coils on top, but it worked and would keep our food from spoiling. It made a nice lulling hum when it was running. It would be perfect for calming a baby.

His friend told him that the pickup had faulty brakes and he should put a rock behind the wheel if he was parking on a hill. To be safe, Kenneth got two big rocks and put them in the pickup. When he got back with his load, he backed the truck up to the porch, and after placing the rocks carefully in front of the wheels, he lowered the tailgate onto the porch floor. Using a borrowed dolly he unloaded everything maneuvered them into the house and put them where I wanted them.

It was almost noon by that time, so he grabbed two oranges, handed one to me, and told me that I should eat something. He was always concerned about my eating habits and would say, "It's for our baby, you know." I started dutifully peeling the orange when he told me to "Get in the pickup. We can return the truck and have lunch when we get back." I climbed in just as he removed the first rock. After I shut the door, he removed the second rock. The truck began to roll and he yelled for me to put my foot on the brake. Looking down, all I saw were peddles. I didn't know which was the brake! He was yelling,"The brake!" as loud as he could, running madly down the hill behind the truck. I didn't drive, so I made a wild guess and jammed my foot down as hard as I could on the peddle closest to me. Nothing happened. He yelled, "Pump it!" I was in an awkward position for pumping. I did my best but nothing was working. That hill was straight down and I was going for the ride of my life, sitting in the passenger seat, stomping on peddles as hard as I could. The truck finally came to a jarring halt. Kenneth grabbed the door open and hauled me out of the pickup.

"Are you okay?" he asked.

"Yes," I said, "but I lost my orange. The darn thing just vanished." I was pretty shaken and was mighty glad to stand on solid ground. Kenneth went around in front of the truck and looked under the front end. When the truck stopped, the bumper was on the road and the front wheels weren't even touching. We sat there on the edge of that hill and marveled at our luck. Kenneth went to the neighbor's and got help to get the truck down on the road. We took it back to the owner and climbed in the Packard for a safe ride home. The first thing we did when we got back to the house was hook up the chimney to the stove. That monster, the blue stove, sat like a Noah's ark in the kitchen. Kenneth had gotten enough stove pipe to connect it to the existing pipe that went through the wall, across the stairwell and into the chimney. After the job was done, I built a fire to warm the place up, grabbed the coffee pot and sat it in place. We were home again. We arranged everything else and put things in the cupboards. Smoke started rolling from the stove. Kenneth adjusted the dampers so it would draw better and we wouldn't become asphyxiated. It never did draw well and to get any heat you had to practically build a bonfire in it.

During the night, it snowed. When I woke up the following morning, I went to the kitchen to start the fire. There was a line of snow clear across the kitchen floor. Then I noticed the door had a crack in it about a half-inch wide from the top, tapering to about a quarter-inch at the bottom. I called Kenneth and we took wads of toilet paper, dampened them and used them to caulk the crack. It worked okay and I hoped it would hold through the rest of the winter. It didn't let us down; it held.

The landlord had a dairy with a large herd of Holstein milk cows. The milk was put in a huge tank in their barn and sent to the creamery every day. They told us that we could buy milk from them and just come to the barn and dip it out of the tank. We got a Quart each day, and because it was Holstein, I had a hard time detecting any cream line. It was not as rich as our cow Betty had given back home but was okay for coffee.

One morning, Kenneth brought the milk and put it in the refrigerator. Usually, by evening, the cream would rise so I could skim a little off for coffee and Kenneth's cereal. I looked at it, and for the life of me, I could not find the cream line. I studied it closely and realized there was no cream line because Kenneth had dipped it so carefully off the top that all he had was cream. When he got home I explained to him that the cream rises and he had to dip deeper so he wouldn't get straight cream. There were several cherry trees in the backyard. I enjoyed seeing the blossoms come on. As they faded, plump juicy cherries began to show themselves. One afternoon, while Kenneth was at work, I sat gazing up into the cherry tree. Luscious big cherries were hanging there, beckoning to me. I picked a few that were hanging low enough to reach, but the most tantalizing ones were up high. I looked at the tree and thought to myself, "I can climb that tree easily." At six months pregnant, I was pretty round but I had climbed my share of trees over the years and this was just a little cherry tree, so up I went, one foot at a time. I picked my cherries and turned to climb down. I got stuck and struggled for at least fifteen minutes and finally freed myself. When I was on the ground at last, I thought how foolish I was. Kenneth wouldn't be home for hours and I could have been stuck all afternoon. I decided that I would not climb any more trees for the remainder of my pregnancy. I sat down and ate my cherries, every one of them.

July 4th was coming up and I was determined to bake a cake. I got up early and built a roaring fire in the stove. Before it had a chance to die down, I popped a cake in the oven. When it came out, it was close to burned on the back, and in the front, it was barely baked and each layer was chisel-shaped. I iced them generously and stacked them so they looked like a cake, almost.

On Sundays, throughout that winter, we'd picked up the local newspaper to read, for after dinner entertainment. I cleaned up the kitchen and we put our chairs on top of the stove with a couple of bricks to put our feet on and read the paper. That was the only way we could keep warm. And, believe it or not, that stupid stove was roaring but gave out very little heat. The stove was so unreliable that Kenneth got some cinderblocks and built a nice barbeque in the backyard. We did a lot of our cooking outdoors and it was very enjoyable through the summer. Life was tolerable and we were young and in love.

Along in late July, Kenneth was outside building a fire in his barbeque, planning on baking potatoes and grilling a couple of small steaks for supper. I had put a fire in the stove to try and heat some water and had really piled on the wood. I looked out the window and thick smoke was rolling by. I heard a crackling sound coming from the living room. Opening the door, I peered in, trying to determine where the noise was coming from. I thought it could be mice. I watched in horror as the wallpaper did a pulsating dance on the wall in the area where the chimney was. I dashed outside, and looking up, saw flames shooting out of the chimney. I yelled,

"Fire!"

Kenneth turned around, took one look and called,

"Go to the neighbor's and call the fire department, and hurry!" I was huge and was at the waddle-only stage of my pregnancy, but boy did I waddle at the same time yelling,

"Fire!" as loud as I could. By the time I got to their house, they had already called the fire company. I turned around and chugged back. When I got there Kenneth was on the roof dumping a bucket of ashes down the chimney. By the time the fire truck got there the fire was out.

When things got tough, Kenneth was a quick thinker. I had no more than started up the hill to the neighbor's than he had grabbed a chain, hooked it to the bumper of the car and threw the other end over the roof right next to the chimney. He hooked the bucket of ashes, which we had by the back door for winter emergencies, over his arm. Grabbing the chain, he literally walked up the side of the house with the bucket of ashes. He dumped them down the chimney, smothering the fire. He, himself could never explain how he did it so fast but the fact is, he did, and he put the fire out.

The problem was that the chimney did not draw properly and, it had accumulated a lot of tar over the years and had never been cleaned.

CHAPTER 7

House #3
Our First Child Arrives

It was time for us to move again, someplace safe, no more hills or bad flues. Good luck smiled on us, we found a nice house next door to the machine shop owned by Kenneth's boss, Bill Case. All Kenneth had to do was walk out the door, take a few steps to the left and he was at work. He could get a little extra shuteye in the morning and come home for lunch. The house had two bedrooms, a large kitchen, a bathroom and a living room that opened onto a full front porch. The basement had the typical 'bucket-a-day' coal furnace. Off the kitchen was a large enclosed porch where we put our refrigerator. The bathroom was big enough to accommodate my washing machine. The kitchen welcomed our big blue monster, the stove which I was actually getting rather fond of. And, bless this house, it had an air conditioner. The summers were hot and humid and this was indeed, a welcome addition. There was a large double-sided desk in the living room, which would be handy. We would have two pieces of furniture in the living room instead of just the hide-a-bed.

There were no closets but Kenneth built a removable closet that we could break down and take with us when we moved. The house was on a dead-end street. At the end was the railroad track, next to the machine shop, our house, an alley, then the First Baptist Church. Behind us was the coal yard and a block down the alley was the hardware store. The parsonage was across the alley from our back yard.

By the end of August, fall was beginning to show her colors and the town was beautiful. Every street was lined with sugar maples and they glowed with color. I got out my watercolors and went to work. It was like a dream come true. I was alive to all the world around me. I painted the church, machine shop, house across the street, leaves, leaves, and more leaves. Every picture had the beautiful trees as the main attraction.

Time flew by and I was getting more and more uncomfortable. September, the magic month, finally arrived. I was more than ready. But nothing was happening. One of Kenneth's co-workers told him to take me for a fast ride on a winding road where there were lots of "howdy-mams." These were places in the road that took a deep dive, down and up. Every weekend we went for rides trying to jar something loose. The 23rd of September was my birthday and I was getting a little anxious but the doctor said, "Your baby will come when it's ready, just be patient." The following day, I began to have a little discomfort. This being my first child, I didn't' have a clue whether it was indigestion or the real thing, so we decided in the afternoon to head for Towanda, where we would be near the hospital. After examining me, the doctor said my time was near but suggested that Kenneth take me to a movie, and after the movie, check in at the hospital. So we went to a movie. I have no idea what it was about or who the actors were. I just wanted to get on with having my baby. We went back to the hospital and checked me in. The doctor mumbled,

"I suppose I should have told you that your water could have broken." That drew a blank. What did he mean by that? By late that evening, Kenneth became a father. The nurse went to tell him that he could meet his little son. As he followed her to the nursery window, there was a slight incline where an addition to the hospital was attached. Kenneth didn't see it and plunged headfirst into the nurse ahead of him. He righted himself and the nurse said,

"Not so fast, Mr. Schwalb. You have plenty of time, 18 years, to be exact." We were parents! Michael Eugene Schwalb was born on September 24th 1951, weight 8 pounds 6 ounces, 21 inches long. We were starting on the most important phase of our journey. Everything had to be done with our little son Michael's future in mind.

I was finally released to go home and start being a real mother. The first few days were a nightmare of feeding, changing, feeding, washing, feeding, changing and lack of sleep. Michael was born hungry and made his needs known in no uncertain terms. I had my Dr. Spock book handy and followed it religiously but could not fill the little guy up. I finally called the doctor and he advised me to give him more water between feedings. This seemed to help or we were getting used to our new routine, whichever. Our son did all the right things at the right times and, of course, we knew he was way ahead of all the other babies in the world. His first smile we documented. Everyone said it was gas but we knew it was a real smile. I pulled his bassinet out in the kitchen so we could marvel at him, and before sitting down to eat, I changed him. He peed in his daddy's coffee. How funny! We documented that. Kenneth picked him up one morning and put him up to his shoulder, patted his little back and he upchucked all over his daddy's shoulder. How gross! Documented that.

When Michael was about three months old, we got suckered into having a kettle party. The company selling the kettles would come to the house and cook a complete meal to demonstrate the wonders of their cooking ware, then serve the meal to your guests, who were supposed to buy tons of kettles. I invited as many neighbors as I had room for, and prepared the house, shining and polishing everything in sight. The day before the party, I checked to make sure everyone I invited would be there. It seems there was a ballgame the evening of the party and everyone canceled out. I was frantic. I couldn't postpone it, so I called Our friends Agnes, Mary Ellen, Dick and Jessie. They all agreed to show up. Whew, what a relief! I was a nervous wreck.

I had everything timed so there could be no hitches, I would give Michael a bowl of Pablum just before everyone arrived and he would be content, I hoped. I went in the pantry and got the Pablum off the shelf at the same time the doorbell rang. I dropped the box of Pablum and it shot out of the box and spread across the floor like the plague.

I never saw anything go so far and so fast. I left it lying there and quickly closed the door as I went to let my guest in. Kenneth saw what happened and, grabbing a broom, disappeared into the pantry. When he came out, the pantry was nice and clean. He looked across the room, catching my eye, and smiled his everything's-under-control smile. I breathed a sigh of relief. My heart swelled with my love for him. I smiled back.

We got through the meal and everyone agreed that it was delicious. Dear old Agnes bought a whole set of kettles. That made my day and I thanked her profusely. I was so relieved to have it over.

Dick and Jessie decided that they had had enough of trying to be farmers and rented the apartment over us. They moved in with their dog Mazy one weekend. Jessie thought it was her duty to act the part of my mother-in-law and began watching me closely, making suggestions now and then when she thought it was needed. As I went about my duties being a mommy. I sang and talked to Michael when he was awake and was enjoying every moment with him. One day, Jessie came downstairs and told me,

"It's really not a good idea to talk baby talk to Michael, because when he starts to say words he won't know the right way to say them. You could cause him to have speech problems." I looked at her and thought, what can I say to keep my place as Michaels mother and not be rude to her, I know she means well.

"Jessie, if you listen closely to how I talk to Michael you will realize that I don't talk baby talk to him, It is 'Mothereeze' which is much different than baby talk and very soothing to a baby. But, I really appreciate your concern." I thought I sounded so learned. Of course she didn't know I had conjured that up on the spot to protect my need to make my own decisions on how to raise my child.

Jessie and I put in a small garden in the backyard and took turns tending it. When the vegetables began to ripen, she would pick them one day and I the next. The tomatoes grew big and plump and I liked to pick them when they were fully ripened. Jessie picked hers when they were barely pink and put them on her windowsill to finish ripening. She got very frustrated with me because I waited so long and told me that I should do as she did. I thanked her for her advice and told her that my mother always told us to pick the tomatoes when fully ripened because they were better for you and I liked them that way. Jessie pondered that a bit and said,

You don't mind if I give you advice, do you?" I smiled and told her that I was very grateful for her friendship and the advice and sometimes it was very useful.

Jessie was fascinated with my washing machine. One afternoon, she came down-stairs and asked me if she could run off a small load of clothes before Kenneth came home. I told her to go ahead. The washing machine was in the bathroom, and after I used it, I let it pump out in the bathtub. It was very handy. After Jessie finished her laundry, she called me from the bathroom.

"How do you empty the machine?"

"Pull the lever on the side but—" and before I could finish telling her to lower the hose into the tub first, I heard her yell. She had pulled the lever with the hose pointing right at her chest. She was soaked from her chest down and she was terrified that Kenneth was going to come home before she got things cleaned up.

"Don't worry," I told her. "Kenneth won't bite. He's pretty tame so calm down." We got things cleaned up and she never asked to borrow the machine again.

One Saturday, when Kenneth was home, we were talking about his mother and father and things they had done together when he was a young boy. He thought they would have been great grandparents. He wished they had lived to see his little son. I reminded him that would happen in its own time and we had to accept what was. Then I said,

"Remember the old saying? If wishes were horses beggars would ride." He laughed and said

"You're right." but I knew that he was missing his parents and it saddened me.

Michael grew and developed new skills almost daily. Turning over by himself, reaching for the mobile I had hung over his crib, and so on. When he was around four months old, we took him to meet Kenneth's Aunt Dorothy and Uncle Walter in New Jersey. I always dressed him in white with blue accents, changing his clothes twice each day even if they appeared clean to the eye. When we went to visit, I made sure that I had the right number of outfits for the numerous changes he would need. Being a new mother, there were some things I had to learn the hard way, such as what happens to a baby sometimes when there is a change in the water you give him. He got diarrhea while at his aunt's and uncle's. I spent most of my time doing laundry and changing him. We left earlier than we had planned, and in a couple of days, he was fine.

The following Friday, we went to Towanda for our routine shopping, and while Kenneth was getting some items that he needed, I took Michael to the five and dime Store to look at the toys. I was wandering down the aisle with him sitting on my arm. I smelled a weird smell and said to myself, "I think plastic has a terrible odor, I wonder why they use so much of it for children's toys." I picked out a shiny red ball for him and handed it to the sales lady. I switched Michael to my other arm to get the money from my purse and saw a strange brown substance running off my arm at the point where he had been sitting.

(Oh! Shit!) "We'll get the ball another time." I said and hurriedly left the store. It wasn't the plastic toys that smelled so bad; it was my shitty little son.

Kenneth found it fun to come home for lunch and have a little time to play with Michael. He got in on teaching him a lot of little games, such as peek-a-boo! and where's Daddy? He would often feed him and just generally connect with him as daddies do.

Coming home for lunch had its drawbacks however. I was not much of a cook but Kenneth liked my tuna fish sandwiches. He made the mistake of telling me that he did and I made him tuna fish sandwiches every day. One noon, looking sadly at his sandwich, he asked,

"Do you know how to make any other kind of sandwich?" Then smiling, he said,

"How about egg for a change?" I boiled some eggs and for the next two weeks, he got egg salad. Poor guy, he got desperate. The next time we went shopping, he went to the deli and got some Leiderkranz cheese, (similar to limburger, just a hair less smelly, but it was bad enough) and a box of crackers. He had cheese and crackers when he came home at noon and seemed to enjoy his lunches more.

Our stove was very handy for Dick and Jessie because it sat right under the register that carried the heat up to their apartment. They not only got the heat from our stove, they also had the advantage of getting heat from our coal furnace. All the registers in the ceilings carried the heat up to their rooms. They never had to stoke the furnaces or buy coal. This arrangement sometimes worked at a disadvantage for them however, because they also got all the smells from our apartment.

One noon, Kenneth came home for lunch and pulled his cheese out of the refrigerator. There was only enough for a taste or two, so he polished it off and went to deposit the paper in the stove, or so I thought. After he went back to work, the smell of cheese permeated the apartment. It seemed to be getting stronger by the minute. I heard the windows upstairs going up. I could not find the source of the smell. It definitely was coming from the stove, however. After eliminating every possible source that I could, I lifted the teakettle. There was the paper from the cheese under the tea kettle quietly filling the air with the aroma of stinky cheese.

When Kenneth came home that evening, he walked in wearing his wicked grin and said,

"Did Jessie come down today?"

"No," I said. "I heard her windows going up, however. I think she packed up and left." We both had a big laugh. I thought I would have to watch him more closely after that shenanigan.

One afternoon, Kenneth told me that he missed the coffee cakes his mother made when he was young and wondered if I could make some for him. I told him that I had never made anything with yeast, if he would help me, I'd give it a try. We got our 'Joy of Cooking' cookbook out and found the recipe for stollen. After making a list of the ingredients, we headed for Dushore to get the items. After supper, that evening, we went step by step through the recipe and by 9 o'clock had our culinary masterpiece ready to pop in the oven. Kenneth had to work the following day, so he went to bed and told me to be sure and not let the Stollen burn. I got a book and sat in the living room to wait. The book was boring and I must have dozed off. I came to when I heard Dick and Jessie upstairs opening windows, lots of them. It sounded like a stampede up there. I sat up into a thick cloud of smoke.

"Oh!! No! My Stollen" I rushed to the oven trying not to breathe, grabbed the coal-black stollen with a pot holder and rushed it outside. When it cooled down enough to touch, I broke it in half. It was charcoal black clear to the core. I opened the windows and went to bed. The next day, I went upstairs and apologized to Dick and Jessie then went downstairs and made a perfect stollen, just to prove to Kenneth that I could. After airing the place out, I washed the curtains and walls; I had to do a complete house cleaning from top to bottom. Another lesson learned. Never try new cooking ideas at night.

CHAPTER 8

Kenneth Gets Hurt at Work And He Goes Hunting

The middle of the following week, I had Kenneth's lunch ready and was watching out the window for his arrival. The door of the machine shop shot open, banging hard against the wall. Two men came rushing out with Kenneth between them, holding his arm in the air. He had a rope tied around his arm and his face was pasty white. Blood was running off his elbow. They jammed him in a car and took off with their tires making an agonizing wail.

One of Kenneth's co-workers came to the door and told me that there had been an accident. Kenneth had gotten hit by a piece of flying metal and fractured his wrist. They were taking him to the doctor in Towanda. I was petrified with fear. I didn't drive and I was stuck with little Michael. We had no phone so all I could do was pray and wait.

About a half an hour went by when the same man came to the door. I was shaking so badly that it was all I could do to stand up. I called for him to come in. He told me Kenneth was patched up and was on his way home. I was so relieved I almost collapsed. Sitting down in the rocking chair, I clutched Michael and rocked. It was not the smooth gentle rhythm he was used to, I was thinking the faster I rocked, the sooner he'd be home.

When he got home, he was still very white. He told me that he had set his machine up and had gone to get a tool. One of the workers thought he had gone home for lunch and opted to borrow his machine.

He took the metal piece out that Kenneth was going to work on, but when he put it back, he forgot to tighten the machine down. When Kenneth came back, he assumed it was as he had left it and turned the machine on. The piece of metal shot out like a piece of shrapnel. He threw his arm up to protect his head. It hit his arm, glancing off and went through two walls, landing in the boss's office. He sat looking shocked and said,

"It's a good thing it didn't hit me in the head I would be gone." I sat down beside him and held his good hand tight. We were very fortunate today; the good Lord was with us for sure. Kenneth was home for a few weeks while he mended. It was nice to have him there and he had the opportunity to have some time with Michael and really interact with him. All too soon, he was back to work but we'd had a chance to tighten our bond a little tighter. He was a wonderful, patient father.

Hunting season arrived and my 'pioneer' husband had to go and 'bag his deer.' I never could figure out why they called it 'bagging.' You sure couldn't get a deer in any of the bags that I had seen. Anyway, Kenneth went to the local hardware store and got a nice hunting vest complete with a pocket on the back to hold 'stuff' in. On the first day of deer season, all the men in town got the day off. They dispersed in every direction while the wives gathered at the post office, or at each other's houses, to exchange news etcetera.

Around four in the afternoon, Kenneth came home and said he had no luck today but would try again tomorrow. He walked coolly through the room. As he passed me, I saw a large bloodstain on the back of his vest. I didn't say a word but put on my 'pretend I didn't see that' act. Kenneth said,

"Would you like to go for a ride? I need to go to Towanda before the court house closes."

Remembering what he had done when he killed the deer on Dick's property a year ago, he would have dressed it out and saved the heart and liver. That would account for the blood on his vest. I knew he had gotten his deer and wanted to surprise me. I was, of course, ready for whatever he had in mind. I never knew what his next act would be. Bundling Michael up for the ride we went to the court house in Towanda. Kenneth went in and got a map. That really puzzled me. Why did he need a map? He studied it for a few minutes, and then we took off for the hills. He found a dirt road that didn't look like it had been used much; it was almost hidden in overgrowth. He turned off the main road and headed back into the hills. After a few miles he turned off onto a smaller road that was barely wide enough to navigate. There were the remains of a fallen house at the end of it. He stopped and got out. Taking out some burlap bags, he laid them across the hood of the car. It was almost dusk and he was getting a little anxious. He told me to come with him, that he would need my help. I made sure Michael was secure. Not far away I saw a pile of tree branches. He removed them and uncovered a dead deer. He was grinning from ear to ear by this time and proud to present his trophy. I helped him get it tied to the car and off we went, heading for home.

On the way home, he explained why he needed the map. He said that he had walked up the mountain and come to the abandoned farmhouse where he had shot the deer. He couldn't find the road he'd come up on and it was too far to carry the deer back to the car. He got the bright idea to get an aerial view of the area to find where the roads went off the main highway back to the old house; It worked: he found his deer. We took it to the local butcher shop to have it prepared for the freezer. The great hunter slept well that night. Not long after that, bear season opened. The machine shop closed for another week so the men could go hunting. Two of the neighbor men invited Kenneth to go with them. They would leave early the first day of the season and planned on being gone for a week. Kenneth gathered his hunting gear and enough food to last the duration. When the big day arrived the three men with all their gear left in the early morning darkness.

I had planned to do a lot of reading, painting, and visiting while he was gone. That was not going to happen. By noon, he was back with a young black bear on his car; he looked bewildered. I looked at him in astonishment,

"What happened?" I asked;

"Well, we got to the campsite and it didn't take us long to set up our camp. Then we were on our way. I stayed down by the road while the two guys went ahead up the mountain to flush out any bears that might be up there when suddenly, i was looking into the face of a young black bear. I instinctively shot, and the bear fell, now I had a bear to take care of. I couldn't leave it for a whole week on the mountain if we were going to eat it, so, here I am, vacations over." He hung the bear on the support post of the clothesline and cleaned it.

The next day, a line of men started coming to my door one at a time to see the bear and tell me their tales of hunting in the woods.

One man told us to get in touch with the local doctor's wife, She had wonderful recipes and knew all there was to know about how to cook bear. After the bear hung for the day, Kenneth took it to the butcher shop to have it cut and packaged. He had them freeze the hide with the head attached, hoping to have it made into a rug. After finding out how much that would cost, he gave it to the butcher. We got in touch with the doctor's wife and learned how to cook bear. It was somewhat like pork, very rich. We had the scrap meat ground and mixed with part beef and seasoned with sausage seasoning. It was very good. Winter was just about over and spring was beginning to show its approach. Little green shoots were coming up out of the soil and the snow had receded into its hiding place to feed the coming spring flowers. We put a length of snow fence up around the front porch to make a safe place for Michael to play. He was crawling well by eight months. Every morning after I finished my chores I took a bucket of warm water with disinfectant and scrubbed the porch floor and the walls as high up as I thought he could reach. Dressed in his warm white corduroy bib overalls and a white sweater, I let him play with the living room door open so he could enjoy the beautiful spring and he was also able to Stay connected with his mama. He loved it.

CHAPTER 9

Robin Is Born

One morning in May I woke up feeling an old familiar feeling. A little nauseated, not bad, but I knew this time what was going on. I was pregnant again. At least, I'd had a little training by now and knew what to expect. Michael was such a good baby that we just knew we were doing things the right way. Kenneth was doing well in the machine shop and his boss thought that in about a year, he would be ready to receive his certificate of completion and be able to work in any factory where his skills were called for. Time seemed to fly through this pregnancy. I was so busy with Michael that I had little time to think about my condition and my anxiety was much diminished. We were looking forward to adding this child to our little family. We formed a closer bond with Our neighbors and had many parties with young married couples who had small children. When I was about three months into my pregnancy, we decided to go on a vacation with our new friends, Bob and Shirley. We had been so busy establishing our lives that we hadn't taken any time off to just relax. Shirley was carrying her third child and was just about as far along as I was. We were both a little round but still pretty active. We chose to go to a little resort in Rhode Island. Bob and Shirley had a big double tent and we planned to stay at a campground for the weekend. One of our other new friends, Betty Kipp, volunteered to take care of Michael. I was hesitant to leave him, but she had two children and was a good mother. Shirley's mother took her two little girls for the weekend. She was fortunate to have her mother living right next door to her and she was always willing to care for her children.

We left New Albany on a Friday evening in July. It was hot and humid, so we left in the evening when it was cooler. Arriving at the campground in Rhode Island, it took only minutes for the guys to erect the tent. We unpacked the prepared food that we had brought for the evening meal and built a campfire to add atmosphere and keep the mosquitoes away. We talked well into the night, and as the fire died down we tucked ourselves in to wait for morning and our first real vacation since we had left Medford.

The following morning, Shirley and I prepared a breakfast of pancakes, bacon and eggs and, of course, Kenneth had brought the coffee pot and had it already perking on the Coleman gas stove we had brought along. After eating, we explored the beach and our surroundings. There was a nice area for swimming, so we donned our bathing suits and went for a midmorning swim.

The men saw fishermen further out on the lake and made a decision to go fishing. We hadn't planned on this, so we had no fishing gear with us. Bob told Kenneth,

"We can get bait at the bait shop and some hooks and string and fish off the boat,". Kenneth agreed, so they rented a boat, got some line, bait and hooks, and we all went fishing. Rowing out to where they seemed to be getting fish, we dropped our lines. Bob started getting bites right away and pulled in a couple of nice fish.

Now you fishermen out there are going to ask me what kind of fish we were getting. Don't ask. I was and am still not a fisher person, so unless it comes from the market with a label, I don't know one from another. I know trout, salmon, and crabs. That's it, so don't ask.

Bob had brought a supply of candy bars that he was munching on, and after the third candy bar, he began to get an upset stomach. He caught another fish then rushed to the back of the boat and lost his breakfast. He made his way back to the front of the boat, pulled in another fish then stumbled to the back of the boat to deposit more of the contents of his stomach in our wake. We had lots of fish, thanks to Bob, but he didn't eat much for the rest of the day.

We had a wonderful weekend and were back home on Sunday evening to pick up Michael from Kipps. He had a bad case of diarrhea, but after being back home for a few days, he was fine.

Michael's first birthday arrived, September 25th and we celebrated with the usual cake and ice cream, letting him mangle the cake before we doled it out, just the three of us. Maybe next year when he understands a little more, we would have a party, but this was so special, we wanted it all to ourselves.

Michael was walking by this time, a little unsteady but he was on his way. I watched him struggling to get himself launched and thought with a smile that this was why they called them toddlers. He would get to a standing position, wave around and take off, then plop, down he would go.

Christmas arrived and for Michael's first Christmas, we outdid ourselves as much as we could afford.

January 1953 and New Year's arrived. I was beginning to feel very uncomfortable. We celebrated New Year's and I waddled around the house, wishing the baby would come. Two more weeks passed and on January 13th- I knew it was getting very close. We had chosen to go to Robert Packer Hospital in Sayre, Pennsylvania this time. I don't remember why but we did. This was going to be a near mistake. We assumed that our new baby would give us plenty of time to make it the seventy some miles that we had to go to get to the hospital. I had a suitcase packed and a lady to watch Michael.

January 14th- I woke up earlier than usual, I had to use the bathroom and my water broke. I called Kenneth. He called the sitter and we were headed for the hospital. I put a folded towel on the seat to protect the car and we sailed out of there. For some reason I started laughing hysterically. Everything about the whole scenario struck me as funny. Poor Kenneth was driving with his neck stretched out toward our goal, as if that would get us there faster. We arrived at the hospital with just minutes to spare. He drove frantically to the emergency entrance. Coming to a screeching halt, he leaped out of the car and hit the ground running. Seeing Kenneth running in his size 13 flat-as-a pancake feet was funny enough, but what happened next was a real crack up.

Not knowing that there were two entrances for patients, one for maternity and one for men, he drove me up to the men's entrance and ran in. Seconds later, he came running out, wild-eyed, leaped into the car and headed for the opposite end of the hospital and another emergency entrance. A nurse with a wheelchair was waiting for me. I was taken in and admitted then rolled into the delivery room just in time to add one more number to the census. A healthy baby boy. Robin Lewis Schwalb, 7 pounds 6 ounces, 21 inches long.

At home, waiting was a cute little pink ruffled bassinet for what was supposed to be my little girl. This little guy was all boy and a born joker. he kept me amused all the time he was growing up. When we got home, I laid him in the little basinet; he looked like a miniature prize fighter in a tutu. I ripped off the ruffles and got some blue-and-white checked material to make a little quilt and put blue trimming around the area where the ruffles had been. This suited him much better.

Michael was absolutely thrilled with his little brother and was by my side anytime I did anything for Robin. One afternoon, I had finished feeding Robin in the living room and laid him in the bassinet for a nap. I went into the kitchen for a minute and left Michael playing on the floor. I went back just in time to catch Michael on the couch. His toes were gripping the couch and he was hanging on to the bassinet as it rolled slowly away from him. With one leap I rescued both babies from a bad tumble. After that, I was more careful and didn't leave Michael in the room alone with Robin until they were older.

At home with two babies, I had my hands full and then some. I finally got a good routine and our little boys were a joy to us. We got a buggy stroller combination that I could put both boys in when I went to the post office. Although Michael was walking, it was easier to keep track of him if I had them both together in one package.

Jessie walked to the post office with me one morning, and a priest that Jessie knew came out of the restaurant and Jessie greeted him. She said,

"Good morning Father," and introduced him to me as Father. Michael was taking this all in, looking very wide-eyed. After the priest went on his way Michael asked,

"Is he my daddy"? He was too young to understand why they called the man Father. I told him

"No. that's his, name. Daddy is your daddy."

Weekends, when Kenneth was home, he spent as much time as he could with the boys. It gave me a chance to do a few things that were impossible to do without help, such as sewing and ironing. One Saturday, I told him that I needed a haircut and didn't know how I was going to find time or space for it. He said I should make an appointment in Towanda the following Saturday and he would take care of the boys, no problem. I was relieved and called for an appointment in the afternoon for the following Saturday.

When the day arrived I prepared an early supper and Kenneth took over, volunteering to clean up the kitchen and take charge of the boys. I was free for several hours. I even had time to do some clothes shopping for myself. After getting my hair cut and styled, I headed for home and my wonderful little family.

I pulled into our driveway and hopped out of the car. Gathering my purchases I went happily into the house calling,

"Mama's home."

I stopped in the kitchen and was struck dumb at the chaos. The table was bare and the dishes, wrapped up in the table cloth, were sitting in the sink. Kenneth called from the living room.

"We're in here." I cautiously peered around the corner into the living room. Kenneth was sitting on the couch with one boy on each side of him. They were, all three, just sitting there.

"What happened?" I asked. He gave me a look that was pure relief.

"Boy, am I glad to see you, you weren't out of sight when Robin dirtied his pants. I went to change him and Michael pulled the table cloth off the table, dishes and all. I got Robin changed but his diaper is in the toilet and I gathered up the dishes and put them in the sink.

Would you like to take over while I go clean up the mess?" I took over and he, fled to the kitchen.

A few minutes later, he stuck his head in the living room and said, "By the way, honey, I forgot to tell you, you look great." He gave me his famous grin. All was well. I thanked him. The boys had really given him the royal treatment, no holds Barred.

CHAPTER 10

Polio

Everything was going well. The boys were healthy, a cold now and then but nothing serious. The summer before Michael turned two, Dick and Jessie moved into a new house that they had built two and a half blocks from us, but on the same street. A young couple, the Hugos, moved into their apartment.

A short while later, we took a little time out for a vacation and went to Rhode Island for a weekend to relax. Michael was just a few weeks short of his second birthday and Robin was almost eight months old. Two days vacation was enough, then back to work on Monday. Michael seemed to be coming down with a cold, and by Wednesday, he was running a slight fever. I put a cot in our room to separate him from Robin, just as a precaution, and gave him extra water and juices. Friday was our day to go shopping, so I called the doctor to have him check Michael. His temperature was back to normal, but I just wanted to be sure that he was okay. I got him up and dressed him. I told him that we were going "bye bye." He was excited and hopped off the cot. He fell down and got up, saying. "Upsy daisy." He took another step and fell again. Concerned, I turned around and told him to,

"Come to Mama." He got up and took one step. His left leg was like a noodle; it did not hold him up. Panic filled my whole being. Grabbing him up, I took him to where Kenneth was waiting, then gently put him down and told him to "go to Daddy." He took one step and down he went. Kenneth picked him up and said, "Get Robin."

I rushed into Robin's room and grabbed him, blankets and all, and we took off for the doctor's office. When we got to the office, we told the doctor our fears. It took him only minutes to send us on our way to the big training hospital in Sayre. We were silent all the way. I felt frozen with fear holding my little son while he chattered away, completely unaware of what was happening to him.

When we arrived at the hospital, they were waiting for us. The doctor had called ahead to let them know that we were coming and what his suspicions were. We were taken immediately to an examining room. I held Michael while they took fluid from his spine. It was painful and he cried out,

"Owie, owie, Mama." It was an effort not to cry out myself, but I talked calmly to him and tried to comfort him as best I could. Kenneth was walking back and forth in the hallway with Robin in his arms. He looked so worried, I wanted to go out and tell him that things were going to be okay, but I didn't even believe that myself. I knew what was happening, Oh yes! I knew.

The doctor was gone for several minutes. When he came back, he took us into a small room and had us sit down. I said to myself; "We are not supposed to be here; we should be shopping." But we were here and we were about to be given some unwanted news. We sat close together, clutching our children, our hopes and dreams scattered in a heap at our feet, our fears hanging like vultures overhead. The doctor spoke the dreaded words,

"Your son has infantile paralysis and will have to be put in quarantine for the accumulated time of seven days. He has already been at home for three, so we'll keep him in quarantine four more days. Then he can be put in the children's ward, where we'll keep him under observation."

Robin woke up and started squirming in my arms. The nurse that was there offered to take care of him until we got Michael settled. I handed him over to her like a robot, not knowing what was going to happen next. Kenneth took my arm and led me out of the room and down to the end of the hall, where he put his arm around my shoulder. He prayed for our little son, asking only that he be able to function in some way and that this terrible disease not spoil his ability to get by in the world. We talked about how we were going to manage to be there for him and still take care of Robin. ROBIN! I had forgotten where the nurse said she would take him until we were ready to go home. I rushed down the hall just as she was going into one of the examining rooms and asked her where he was. She said,

"He's right here and I will stay with him until you are ready to go, so please don't worry." I thanked her. Then the doctor came and told us that they were taking Michael to the quarantine ward on the third floor and I was welcome to come with him. They didn't know how close I was going to stay to him but they would find out soon enough. We went to the third floor and they rolled Michael into a large room about the size of our school gymnasium. There were only two cribs in the room. It was so empty and big that even the air seemed to echo.

In one corner was a sink with a small table beside it. A stack of paper towels and a box of rubber gloves sat neatly on the table. By the table was a waste container, empty and clean. He would be all alone in this big cold room. I had no time to waste. I had to get Robin home and settled and get back here as soon as possible. The nurse tucked Michael in and told me that I had to stay 10 feet from the bed. I could talk to him from that distance, but I was not to pick him up or touch anything in the room but the chair that I was allowed to sit in.

Kenneth stood outside the door and waited for me to get Robin from the nurse three floors down. I told Michael,

"Bye bye, Mama will be back pretty soon." I threw him a kiss and hurried out. Kenneth was already heading down with Robin when I caught up with him. My mind was thinking of all the possibilities of finding someone to take care of Robin. Then I remembered a woman that went to the church whose daughter had polio a few years ago. She had no other children. Maybe we could recruit her to take care of Robin until Michael was out of quarantine. I told Kenneth about her and suggested we talk to her.

"It's worth a try," Kenneth said. "Let's go, so you can get back here."

We got home around 9 p.m. and called the woman that I had mentioned. She said she would be glad to help and told me to bring his things over. She even had a crib that she had kept, hoping some day to have another child. She turned out to be an angel and so good with Robin.

After getting him settled, I packed a suitcase planning to stay at a rooming house across from the hospital. Kenneth said that he would look in on Robin every day while I was gone. The woman who was caring for Robin told Kenneth to plan on having his meals with them for as long as he liked.

We left and headed straight back to the hospital. It was a long sad drive. When we got there, I checked into the rooming house, kissed Kenneth and told him to try not to worry and to think positive. We would get through this. He said that he loved me and to take care of myself and we parted. I walked across the street to the hospital and climbed the stairs to the big swinging doors and went inside. As the doors closed behind me, from somewhere on the upper floor, I hear a child crying. I listened for a moment then realized it was Michael. I didn't bother with the elevator but took the stairs on the run two at a time, two flights up. As I got closer, the crying became louder and more insistent,

"MOMMY! MOMMY!" I got to the room, and shot in the door. To heck with the rules, my child needed me. He was on the floor under the crib: the side of the crib had been left down and he could not get up. I scooped him up in my arms, telling him, "Don't cry Mommy's here." I sat down with him in the rocking chair and comforted him, promising not to leave. He finally settled down a little, then, all hell broke loose. A doctor and two nurses arrived out of breath, flustered, to say the least, and full of excuses. One nurse said she had given him some prunes and he must have slipped out of bed when he tried to get a prune pit that had fallen on the floor. I asked her who had left the side of the crib down but she didn't have an answer. The doctor told me that I was breaking the rules; I could not touch my son. I told him I would put him in his bed when he felt safe and I wanted a lounge chair because I did not intend to leave the room for one minute. The other nurse that had come in asked me if I would like a cup of coffee. I told her I would. The doctor looked Michael over and determined that there were no injuries and asked me to please follow the rules on using the paper towels to turn the water on and off when using the sink and not to touch the door handle without the paper towel. I agreed and a lounge chair arrived along with a pot of coffee. I had never had coffee but I drank the whole pot, black. I didn't close my eyes for twenty-four hours: I was like a zombie, wound up and moving. I settled down in the chair and sang to Michael until I knew he was asleep. I sat all night with my thoughts on my family. I prayed for strength with every fiber of my being.

Saturday morning dawned early. They brought Michael's breakfast, and while the nurse fed him, I went to the rooming house and grabbed a Danish roll and a cup of coffee, took a hasty shower and ran back to the hospital as fast as I could get there. The doctor came in and told me that he had gotten enough of the Salk vaccine to give to both Robin and me as a protection from the disease. We found out this serum had been available for some time but they were only using it in trial areas. Kenneth's nephews were fortunate enough to live in New York, which was one of the trial areas. I asked myself, "Why Michael? Why us?" God only knew. I called Kenneth via the neighbors because we still didn't have a phone. I told him to bring Robin that afternoon to get the shot. He arrived around two and I had him take Robin in. So my little Robin got the protection from this terrible thing, and I was next. The doctor said because of his age, Kenneth would, likely not be affected.

The serum was given so many c.c.'s per pounds of body weight and I was a little on the chunky side. I got two shots, one in each hip. I felt as if I had been kicked by a mule, twice. That's what I told the nurse when she asked me why I was limping.

I spent the remainder of the day playing games, reading, and generally entertaining Michael. When he was taking his nap, I took advantage of the time to grab a nap for myself.

That Sunday afternoon, a frightened little six-year-old girl was brought in. She was given a bed close to the door and her mother told me that she was there for observation; she didn't have the paralysis as yet, but she had other symptoms. She was very quiet. Her mother told her she would go down and get her a book and she must remain as quiet as she could until she got back. She left and was gone all day. The poor child waited and waited. She finally asked me when her mother was coming. I told her I didn't know, maybe she had some errands to run. I created some fun guessing games to help keep her Occupied, and her mother never came back until Monday. It was all I could do to hold my tongue, I thought, what a terrible way that was to treat a child.

Monday evening I was allowed to feed Michael and he ate as usual. He was always a good eater. After supper, we played games and I told the children stories with as much animation as possible to amuse them. That evening, after singing them to sleep, I finally dozed off myself and slept through the night until around 5 a.m. I rushed over to the rooming house to take a shower and grab a bite of breakfast and hurried back in time to be there when they brought Michael's breakfast. The orderly sat it on the small table by his crib. I lowered the side so I could feed him better and sat him up. He flopped over like a rag doll. He was completely paralyzed; he couldn't even hold his head up. I was devastated but managed to stay calm and called the nurse. She told me this was normal for this disease and he would probably start coming out of it by Monday. She also told me it was alright to hold him on my lap and hold his head up for him. They had finally given up telling me that I couldn't touch him.

Thank God, the nurse was right. By Tuesday, he was sitting up again and by Wednesday, he was pulling himself up to stand in the crib, but he was not using his left leg at all. That Afternoon, the doctor put a cast on his leg to keep him from using it. He needed to observe him to see where the damage would localize. Michael was now able to go to the children's ward and would not be so alone.

It was September 25th, his second birthday. Kenneth brought a little cake and we sang Happy Birthday to him and gave him a silly rubber ball with a face on it, which when squeezed, stuck out its tongue. It terrified him so badly that we had to get rid of it. This concerned me, he had never shown fear of anything before. I didn't want him developing psychological problems on top of everything else. I made a note to talk to the doctor about this.

The mothers of the children in the ward formed a pact. We would take turns being with the children, just to talk to them and basically keep them from getting lonely and scared. I took a break and went home to connect with Robin and Kenneth. Every other day, I went to be with Michael. The doctor didn't tell us how long he would be there, but we kept hoping some good would come of it. A couple months went by and I was getting used to going back and forth. Leaving Robin with his sitter. Around noon, I would head for the hospital armed with new books and toys to share with Michael and the other children in the ward.

One afternoon, I got there before nap time was over. The room was dark, and most of the children were asleep. I heard a quiet sobbing; tiptoeing up to Michael's crib, I looked at him lying on his tummy, sobbing in his sleep. He had diarrhea and his crib was a mess from end to end. He had on a pair of men's briefs. I knew from the sound of his sobbing that he had been crying hard before he had fallen asleep. His little face was swollen and red. I took one look and reaching under his bedside table I grabbed the wash basin. After filling it with warm water from the bathroom, I cleaned him up. The more I Cleaned, the angrier I felt. What kind of a place was this to do such a thing to a child?

After I got him clean, I went to the closet where I knew the diapers were kept. The shelf was bare. I took a nice clean blanket and wrapped him up then marched out of the room with my son in my arms. As I walked by the nurse's station, I said, without stopping,

"I'm taking my son home. Have him checked out by the time I get down to the checkout station." The nurse finally came alive;

"Oh, Mrs. Schwalb you can't do that. The doctor hasn't released him."

"That's okay" I told her, "I'll bring him back every day if necessary, but he is going home where he'll get better care." I kept on walking down to the checkout. I was determined that they were not going to stop me. I took Michael home. The doctor made an appointment for weekly visits and we were once again a family.

Home again, what a relief. I had a list of exercises that Michael was to do daily and a whole book of rhymes to say as he did them. He had been in the hospital for two and a half months. When he got home he thought he could do things like before, and when he couldn't, he would throw himself on the floor and scream,

"I tan't walk!" I waited for him to calm down and then said,

"Let's crawl like Robin." I got down on the floor and crawled as fast as I could, making a game of it. I hid behind the couch and called for him to find me. When he did I chased him so he had to crawl fast to get away from me. He squealed with laughter and Robin got into the game. We crawled all over the house until we were all exhausted. On the first week's scheduled trip back to the doctor we waited in the waiting room while the other children waited their turns with their mothers.

Children were demanding and throwing temper tantrums when they didn't get what they wanted. Michael was taking all this in. I watched him concentrate on their actions while the mothers were trying to appease their children. I said to myself,

"Oh no you don't, young man. I will not give in to temper tantrums" and I never did. He was not prone to temper tantrums as long as I helped him find a solution to what was bothering him.

The doctor did not want him to stand on his leg yet, so he put him in night braces. His shoes had metal plates on the soles with a flat bar attached to each shoe, keeping his feet bound together. He could stand but could not walk. He had to wear them day and night. This was also supposed to keep his leg and foot from twisting as he grew.

Michael hated the brace, so I taught him to crawl with both knees coming forward at once, like a little rabbit hopping. I got some leather coat sleeve patches to put on the knees of his pants and he was free to travel as much as he wanted.

Every week for a month, we kept our appointments with the doctor. He finally told us that we would only need to come once a month. Winter was coming and it was a big relief not to have to make that long trip when the snows came. We kept up the exercises and he seemed to be making progress in some areas but the left leg remained useless. We did get some action in his hip however.

CHAPTER 11

Bells Palsy

Fall was advancing with her beauty and the leaves were beginning to come down, covering the ground with gold; they were irresistible. Kenneth raked up a big pile one Saturday and took both boys out to play in them. They came in all rosy-cheeked and ready for supper.

After we had eaten, Kenneth bathed the boys while I cleaned the kitchen. I heard him reading to them, then all was quiet and we had the evening to ourselves. We didn't talk much about what had happened to Michael, but we did talk of things we could do to make his life as normal as possible. We knew he didn't need his leg to use his brain and that seemed to be doing just fine. He was a big boy for his age and seemed to be ahead in years. His speech was developing well and he was full of questions about his surroundings. He was a bright, inquisitive little boy and never complained about his leg but took it in stride as if it was natural.

Michael's third birthday was approaching and we decided to get him a tricycle to encourage him to use his legs when the doctor took the night braces off. A few days before his birthday, he started running a fever and the side of his face was swollen. I called the doctor. He said mumps were going around and Michael was probably getting them. He suggested keeping him out of drafts and pushing fluids, which I was already doing. Two days later, Robin woke up screaming and pulling on his ear. I took him to the doctor, who examined him and found that he had an infected ear. He gave him a shot of penicillin. It was his assumption that Robin was coming down with the mumps and would probably have more problems with his ear. That didn't happen: his ear was fine in a few days and he never got the mumps.

Michael got worse, however. I called the doctor again and he told me that Michael was having a harder time getting over the mumps and I was to push the fluids and wait it out.

When I went to bed, I left the boys' door open so I could hear every little squeak from their room. I slept very lightly, getting up several times to check on them. Before we went to bed, I had Kenneth bank the fire in the kitchen stove, which was just outside the boys' room. I always left a teakettle full of water on to keep moisture in the air. A couple days went by and Michael was still not getting better. The third night, I went to bed and slept for about four hours. I woke up suddenly, hearing an unfamiliar sound coming from the kitchen. It sounded like something cooking on the stove, like bubbling cereal. I couldn't make it out, so thought I had better investigate. I went into the kitchen but there was nothing on the stove. The sound was coming from the boys' room. I turned on the light and was totally shocked at the sight before me. Michael was lying on his back on his little bunk bed. His face was covered in blood. It was bubbling like a fountain from his nose. He was wearing his little sleepers with the feet in them. The blood had seeped down to his waist and was soaking the sheets to the edge of his bed. Grabbing him up, blankets and all. I rushed to the bathroom. I had to get the flow of blood stopped. Laying him in the bathtub, I called Kenneth to go to the public phone on the corner and call the doctor. Then I told him,

"Don't come in, Michael has a very bad nosebleed." Kenneth had a problem when he saw anyone bleeding. He would sometimes pass out and I really needed him right then. I grabbed two trays of ice from the refrigerator. As I ran warm water in the tub to keep Michael warm, I got a towel and filled it with ice, packing it around his head, concentrating on getting it on his temples. Somehow, I was able to stop the bleeding, but he was as white as paste and limp as a rag. I sat with him cradled in my arms and prayed, "Dear God, not again." Kenneth came back and said

"The doctor wants to see him first thing in the morning." I sat up the rest of the night with Michael. When morning came, I whipped around as fast as I could and got him to the doctor.

What had happened was the main artery on the right side of his face had become infected. It was not mumps; it was an infection. It finally burst, causing him to hemorrhage, it left the right side of his face paralyzed. He had Bell's Palsy. The doctor gave me three tiny white pills to give him, one each night when I put him to bed. He said that Michael would have more nose bleeds but they would gradually stop.

That evening, I took the little cot in our room and put it beside my bed and sat with him until he went to sleep.

Kenneth cleaned up the kitchen for me and put Robin to bed. Michael had eaten a good supper and seemed to feel fine but I was taking no chances. When I went to bed, I pulled his cot up close to my bed and laid my hand just in front of his nose so I could feel him breathe. I was that worried. He slept soundly until around two o'clock when he began to stir. I turned on the light and his nose was bleeding again, but not so badly I was able to stop the bleeding right away. I sat and watched him for a while until he went back to sleep, then got a few winks myself until it was time to start my day. Kenneth was up early and had the coffee made. He had a cup ready for me and offered to fix my toast.

"How's Michael doing?" he asked.

"He seems to be better," I told him. "I hope that this is going to be a good day for him." We sat and talked for a few minutes until he had to leave for work and it was time for me to get the boys up.

Two more nights and two pills later, Michael seemed to be okay again, feeling fine and playing with Robin. The doctor put him on an iron-rich diet. He told me to give him liver at least once a week. Michael was not fond of liver, so I made German liver dumplings which he loved. I ground the liver and mixed it with softened bread crumbs, added some chopped onion, parsley, a sprinkle of salt with two tablespoons of flour, beat two egg whites and blended them with the mixture. I dropped spoon-size balls into simmering soup stock and cooked them until they were firm. Michael loved these little balls of liver, I put molasses in his milk and gave him raisins to snack on.

CHAPTER 12

Kenneth Finishes His Training

Fall had come with a flurry of orange, red and gold to brighten our days. Kenneth and the boys had many happy Saturday afternoons playing in the leaves, and then the leaves became tired and crumbled away to make way for the first snow. Kenneth came home one Friday evening with a big grin on his face and said "Tonight I want a nice juicy steak with all the trimmings." and handed me a big envelope. I pulled out a large white important-looking certificate that said,

"CERTIFICATE OF COMPLETION OF APPRENTICESHIP" with his name written on it in large fancy lettering-

KENNETH A.SCHWALB—smack dab in the middle and two large gold seals on each side at the bottom. He was ready for anything that he chose to do in his field. The next step was to find a factory where he would get good wages and benefits. I gave him a big hug and fixed him a steak with all the trimmings, you bet I did!

Sunday after church, we got the paper and started looking through the "help wanted" sections, writing down names and addresses. Kenneth had a list of good factories that his boss, Bill Case, had suggested. He thought he would write to them first and try to Get interviews. One place his boss thought would be good to start was a factory in Buffalo, New York. It was quite a distance but it sounded promising. They offered good benefits, had very few strikes and layoffs, and the pay was good.

Kenneth wrote to them. A couple of weeks went by before he got an invitation to come for an interview. We chose the very next weekend to go. It was winter and snow was still piled here and there in dirty, slushy piles, but the roads were clear and well cindered.

Leaving early in the morning with enough supplies to last the day, we arrived in Buffalo a little after noon. While Kenneth went in for his interview, I gave the boys the lunch that I had packed for them. The snow was piled high along the sidewalks, and in some places, it was higher than the cars. I thought to myself, "They must have some pretty wild snow storms here."

After about an hour, Kenneth came out smiling. He had gotten the job and was to report for work in two weeks. Our spirits were soaring as we drove home making plans. I would have to get Michael's medical files transferred and have his doctor connect me with a doctor in Buffalo. Kenneth said that he would get a room the first week and look for a place for us to live and move us the first weekend so we wouldn't be separated long.

On Monday, Kenneth went to work and gave them his two weeks notice. The guys at work had a little party for him, congratulating him and wishing him well. The next two weeks flew by. We did some packing so we wouldn't have it all to do at the last minute. I told Michael's doctor what to expect. He said that he would transfer his papers when we got settled. The time was gone before we knew it and the day arrived for Kenneth to leave. He had clothes packed to last a week, a few groceries and, of course, the coffee pot. It was time to say goodbye. We hugged him and waved as he drove away to our future.

It was a long day, but I had plenty to do and the time went fast. After the boys were tucked into bed, I got a book and sat in the living room for awhile. It was getting dark outside but there had not been any new snow during the day and it was a clear night.

As I sat reading, I heard something on the porch like someone walking. I peered out the window. It was Kenneth. I grabbed open the door and said,

"What happened?" He was crying. I had never seen him so distressed.

"I didn't pass their physical," he replied, "They turned me down. I have a hernia." He came in the house and sat down with his head in his hands. I sat beside him and said,

Honey, don't worry. Things will work out." He said, "Dolores, you don't understand. I've quit my job so I can't draw unemployment and nobody is going to hire me with medical problems."

We sat and talked for a long time, and at last, we decided that the best thing for him to do would be to go ahead with the operation. I would get part-time work until he was ready to go back. We could never go forward as long as he put it off.

Kenneth went to the doctor the following day and got scheduled for his operation. I was pretty thrifty, so we had enough money set aside for a few weeks, but with Michael still going to the clinic every month, it wouldn't last long, no matter how frugal I was.

When Kenneth got home after the operation, the doctor said he could do no lifting or straining for three months.

I was strong and healthy and perfectly able to do anything that he couldn't do, so when he was well enough, we did some switching of chores. He did light housework for me and watched the boys, and I went out looking for small part-time jobs. I told my friends about our situation, and that I would be open to any small jobs they may have. Mae Waltman was papering a lady's house and she asked me if I would paint the woodwork in the living room. That brought in a little money. Then I did a mural on the wall of another lady's new house. Here and there, I got enough work to keep us going. One afternoon, there was a little league ball game at the school and I grabbed my watercolors and went to the game. Sitting on the bench behind the screened area, I painted character pictures of the boys playing ball. The parents thought that was fun. I sold the pictures for five dollars apiece and had a little enjoyment at the same time. We struggled along for a couple of months. Then Robin got a bad cold. We barely had enough gas to get us to Towanda to the doctor and back home again. Kenneth said,

"Dolores, I know how hard you are trying, but I don't think we're going to make it. We're behind on our electric bill and the rent is due. I can't tell Bill that I won't be able to pay the rent. He's been so helpful;

that would be wrong. I'm afraid we're going to have to ask for help." This was a real shock, I had never in my life asked for help and neither had my parents. We had always found a way, no matter what. I felt defeated but I knew he was right. We applied for assistance. Our first check came two weeks later, the day we took Michael to the clinic. On the way through Towanda, we stopped to pay the doctor what we owed him for treating Robin's cold and cashed the check there, got gas and went on to Sayre to the clinic. When we had applied for assistance they had taken a lot of information from us, including my parent's name and address. I had no idea that they would get in touch with them but a check came in the mail from my mother. I couldn't believe it. Never in all my life had I ever asked for money or borrowed from anyone, especially not my parents. I was humiliated beyond belief. I didn't even want them to know we were having trouble. I sat down and wrote a long letter to her thanking her for the check and told her that I was sending it back because we didn't need it. Kenneth would soon be ready to go back to work and we were doing just fine. I thanked her again and told her that I would write when we had some good news" Don't worry, Mama. We're okay." I told her I had a good mama that taught me how to survive and that I loved her. It was two more weeks before Kenneth was released to go back to work. He wasted no time and found a job with Westinghouse in Nicholson, Pennsylvania. It was much closer than Buffalo, New York. Which I was thankful for.

CHAPTER 13

We Move to Nicholson

We moved to Nicholson, Pennsylvania next door to a man who worked at the same place where Kenneth would be working. They were able to take turns driving, which cut down on the gas, which was a big help.

The house we moved to was a big square two-story Colonial with a full basement. The kitchen was attached. A flagstone entry led to the kitchen. There was no running water, which meant back to the outhouse again. There were two kitchens. One was a working kitchen with a pitcher pump and a tin sink. To those who don't know what a pitcher pump is, it is an iron pitcher-shaped item with a handle that is pumped up and down to draw water up from a well. A large milk can sat in the corner for extra water. There were two walls of cupboards with real marble countertops. We put our big blue stove in the other kitchen where we would eat.

Off the kitchen was a dining room. Beyond the dining room was the living room. Upstairs were three bedrooms. The master bedroom had a small room off to the side where we put the boys. The third bedroom we used for storage.

We brought all our small items in, then got the boys' beds set up. We borrowed Bill Case's truck to move the stove, couch, bed and another small couch that we had acquired from a neighbor. Not much furniture for a big house, but we spread it out and it was fine. My house cleaning would be simple.

It was so cold the day we moved that when we got back with the second and final load, the milk sitting on the counter was frozen, the cream standing up a good inch out of the bottle. We hooked up the stove and went to the basement to build a fire in the furnace. The floor was clean and shiny, although it was dirt, it looked like concrete. I wondered how the little old lady who had lived there previously had kept it so clean. When we had gone to pay her the rent, she opened the door and I was shocked to see how tiny she was. She was bent almost double. I could not imagine a woman like her keeping a house that big clean with no help. She had lived there with her husband, caring for him until he passed away, and then she had decided to move to a small apartment where she wouldn't have so much housework. She gave me some housekeeping tips on how she had kept the place so clean. She said;

"Every morning, I go to the basement with my broom and a bucket of water. I dip my broom in the water and sprinkled the floor then sweep it, the drying earth along with the soft touch of the broom gives it the shine that makes it look like concrete."

The outhouse had beautiful white wallpaper on the walls, generously covered with big red roses. A small shelf in one corner had a white-enameled bucket half full of lime. Above it, hanging on a nail, was a long-handled dipper. After each use, she told me to sprinkle a dipper of lime in the regions below. This would keep it clean and odor-free. I thought of my childhood and how I hated the smell of the outhouse. I never dreamed there could be a solution.

Water was going to be our biggest problem. Down a long path behind the house off to the right was a spring, much like the one I had grown up with in Oregon. The water was sweet, clear and very cold coming from deep in the earth. But it had to be carried because we found out the pump in the kitchen did not work anymore for unknown reasons.

We were approximately one mile from town, and upon entering, we passed the local creamery. Kenneth asked them if we could get water for laundry on the weekends. They gave us permission to do so on Saturday mornings. Kenneth got several cans of hot water that filled my washing machine and two tubs. After washing the clothes, I dried them in my new automatic drier. I felt as if I were living in two separate time zones. There was no bathtub and the sink was too small to bathe the boys in. We needed a place for Michael's water exercises. We went to the local hardware store and bought a watering trough that was meant to be used for cattle. We used it for a bathtub for all of us. Sitting it on the back porch by the washing machine, we created a bathroom. Hooking a hose up to the drain, we were in business. During the summer, Kenneth and I went to the spring late in the evening for bathing in the runoff. It was cold but adequate. We felt like pioneers.

Spring was coming and I was excited to see things pushing up through the earth trying to bloom. There was a tangle of rose bushes in an area where trash had been dumped. The first thing I did was to clean up that particular spot to make the yard safe for the boys to play in. I uncovered a wonderful sunken rose garden with a flagstone floor about ten feet in diameter. It was lush and thick with roses of all colors. Its beauty gave me a tranquil place to sit on occasions just to rest.

While cleaning up the yard, I found another dumping place on the bank behind the outhouse. I cleaned that up also, finding many useful treasures. One item was a barrel stave churn complete with a wooden dash. I carefully cleaned it with a wood preservative, got a length of iron pipe that I painted black, and made a nice standing lamp to sit beside my couch. I then bought a burlap shade that was perfect for it. I felt so smart that I started looking for other items I could find uses for.

The house was on a hill and down at the back of the house was a barn that looked like it hadn't been used in years. One afternoon, when the boys got up from their naps, I took them down to explore the field and barn. There were wild strawberries everywhere we walked. Of course we had to sample them on our way. When we went in the barn, it was not spooky like the barn I remembered from my childhood, but wide open and friendly with the sun pouring through the cracks and areas where boards were missing. There was a loft with a sturdy ladder built in. I couldn't resist; I had to check it out. Up I went with the boys wide-eyed, watching me. To my utter surprise, there, carefully placed, was a flax wheel complete with flax still attached. There were two unfinished maple twin beds, a wonderful well-used tub bench large enough for two tubs, a Pennsylvania Dutch batter pitcher and some stoneware pie dishes, crocks, a few enameled items and two large wooden bowls. One was round and the other was a large rectangular one that I later found out was used to knead bread in and was known as a bread trough. What a find! For the next few afternoons the boys and I toted things to the house.

When we went to pay the rent, I asked the elderly lady about the items. She told me they had been put there many years before and I was welcome to them.

The boys and I spent many happy hours in this wonderful old house. Each day after Kenneth left work and my housework was done, we explored until noon, then I fed the boys their lunch, and after reading to them, put them down for their naps. They slept for about an hour, then were up to explore on their own.

One afternoon, I noticed some unusual things hanging in the trees; they looked like miniature tents. Kenneth told me they were caterpillar tents and the caterpillars would soon be coming out of them. I showed them to the boys and they were fascinated as they watched for the caterpillars' entry into the world. When they finally came out, Robin was especially excited because they were fuzzy like his teddy bear. I would see him playing outside with a few caterpillars gathered up, stooping down talking to them and gently brushing them with the tip of his finger. One afternoon, he came inside and was playing on the couch. When I called him to supper, he left his sneakers sitting by the couch. While he was eating, I noticed them there and put them in the closet. After he finished eating, he ran back in the living room and called to me,

"Mama!" I went to see what he wanted and he asked,

"Where's my shoes?" I told him that I put them in the closet. He rushed over to the closet, tugged the door open and grabbed his shoes. Looking up at me he asked,

"Where are my wittle wo'ms?" He had filled his shoes with Caterpillars, I found about a dozen of them in the couch.

Robin was a very sensitive little boy and liked everything to run smoothly. Michael was always exploring and sometimes this got him a scolding. We had some friends drop by for a visit and I asked them to have tea with us. I put the teakettle on the stove to heat, and when it was boiling, I fixed the tea. When I poured the water, a red oily substance came out. Michael had put a red crayon in the tea kettle. I rushed around and heated water in a sauce pan and made the tea. After the guests left, I scolded Michael for putting the crayon in the kettle and told him never to do that again and had him repeat what I said. Robin stood watching wide-eyed and concerned. Then he ran to his toy box and got his favorite book, *Filbert the Donkey*. In the story, Filbert ate the flowers off the Mayor's wife's hat and was put in a shed with a lock on it. There's a picture of Filbert locked up and crying. Robin found the picture and buried his face in the book and began crying loudly, saying,

"You scolded my brudder." Then he wailed until I promised not to do that again. I told him,

"I'm not mad at your brother. Mama just wants him to learn to do nice things because Mama loves your brother."

CHAPTER 14

Robin Has His Tonsils Out And The Boys Meet Their Grandparents

Robin had a few colds that always ended with a sore throat and the doctor decided he should have his tonsils removed. He was three years old and we had very few problems with him with the exception of the sore throats. On the day of his appointment, I left Michael with our neighbors, who offered to care for him for the three days Robin would be hospitalized. They had two children our boys ages and she was a careful mother so I was comfortable with this arrangement. The doctor assured me that this was a pretty routine operation, but all operations carried some risk.

On the scheduled day, I took Robin in. When the doctor told him that he wanted to stick his finger, Robin held his little finger out and the doctor stuck it; Robin didn't budge. They put him on a gurney and wheeled him down the hall. I went into his room to wait. Another mother was waiting for her child to come back. Her little girl was scheduled to have her tonsils removed after Robin. We chatted and in no time the orderly was back with Robin still under anesthesia. The orderly picked him up and laid him on his bed. He said,

"He was the best little guy. He did everything we asked without a whimper," Then he smiled and walked out of the room. I looked at Robin who was peacefully sleeping. He took a deep breath and suddenly stopped. It sounded as if he'd swallowed a cork. He was not breathing. I looked at him for a frantic moment, realizing that his tongue had gone down his throat. I screamed loudly to the mother who was waiting for her child.

"GET A NURSE, FAST!" I knew I had to get Robin's mouth open. There was a stack of five tongue depressors on the table taped together. Grabbing them I and tried to pry his mouth open. His jaws were locked and he was turning blue. Managing to get the tongue depressors between his teeth I twisted them as hard as I could. They broke apart in my hand. I thought to myself that I would have to break his jaw if necessary to get his mouth open. I pulled his head over the side of the bed to elongate his throat, hoping that it would relax his tongue, then thrust my fingers in beside his teeth. I was making headway when a very pregnant nurse came running in with an oxygen machine. Together we got his mouth open and she hooked him up to the machine. He began taking big noisy gulps of air and his color came back. I collapsed. I was shaking so badly that I could not stand up. I stayed with him the three days he was there. Every time I looked at him, I thanked God that I had been there at the right time. The day Kenneth came to take us home, I went to the gift store downstairs and bought a teddy bear that became Robins Constant companion until he went off to school, and even then he included his bear in show-and-tell at school and at summer camp any time he could.

Two summers before when Robin first started to walk, we had taken our first trip back to Oregon to visit my parents. At last the boys would get to meet their grandparents. There were no words in the English language to tell how elated I was. I would be bringing the biggest joy of my life home to show my parents. I knew that we had the most delightful little boys a grandparent could wish for. We would camp along the way and show some of the sights to the boys. Whether they would remember them was another thing.

The trip went smoothly until we were in the middle of desert country and noticed small items missing—Kenneth's handkerchiefs, one at a time, Robin's shoes. We soon found the leak. Robin was blazing his own trail, dropping items out the window at regular intervals across the West. We stopped somewhere in Wyoming to get a pair of Moccasins for him. I watched him more closely after that.

One noon, we found a campground along the river, and we stopped to have lunch. After we ate, I took my little bucket of soiled diapers down to the river to wash them. There were big bushes here and there. I looked up and saw a group of people with cameras looking down on me. I stood up to see what was going on and looked across the bushes into the face of the biggest moose I had ever seen. I got out of there in a hurry, and after that, I watched for wild animals anytime I left the car.

The closer we got to Oregon, the more anxious I got. I had prepared a lunch of sandwiches and fruit for our last stop before we got to Medford. When we stopped, I laid out our lunch as fast as I could and was ready to go. Then Kenneth decided to shine his shoes for his grand entrance. My stomach was in a knot. When we finally made it to Medford and drove up in my parents' yard, I was bawling like a baby.

My dear parents, they were the same as when I had left them and were more than ready to spoil our little sons. The first thing Mama did was get them some Western "Levi" jeans. Next came the,

"What, they've never had candy?" Mama said, "We'll fix that." The boys were launched into the real world. Grandmas and grandpas became special people in their book.

Robin was just beginning to walk and we were waiting for his first word. He would manage to get himself to a standing position, then lose his balance and plop down on his bottom. He was in the kitchen and had managed to struggle to a stand when he suddenly did his plop and finished with his first word,

"Nuts." Not "Daddy" or "Mama," but a clear, plain, "nuts." That was Robin. He did things differently all of his life. Our neighbor, Mrs. Stauffer, came over to visit and Michael climbed up on the couch beside her. He was a friendly little boy and loved meeting people. She dubbed him "a lovable teddy bear." He came back with, "I'm not a bear, I'm a boy."

All too soon, it was time to go home, but our mission was accomplished. Now I knew I would be able to go home now and then. In the following years, I still would get very homesick but this trip would help me pull myself out of it, knowing that I could and would see them again.

CHAPTER 15

Michael Has His First Surgery And Christmas in Nicholson

The fall of 1955, Michael turned four. He had his first corrective surgery to help him to eventually get out of the braces. They measured his legs every time we went to the clinic, and when he got to a certain growth development, the doctor decided to put a bone extension in his leg. This consisted of separating his shin bone and inserting a piece of dead bone from the bone bank. He explained to me that this would eventually take life from the living bone and grow along with it. At the same time, he used a piece of living bone from Michael's shin as a shim under his ankle to straighten his foot that was turning to the outside. This all worked fine but he still had to wear the brace. The operation was done over the holidays and Michael was in the hospital for only two weeks.

After Thanksgiving, Christmas was on the horizon. Kenneth was having a great time with the boys. The autumn leaves had been played in and put to rest. The snow had come gently at first then in silent cascading urgency to pile up in the yard. It seemed as though every day I shoveled snow. It was so beautiful; I loved being out in it. One morning after Kenneth went to work, I was in a hurry to get my chores done and grabbed the snow shovel, shoveling as fast as I could and lifting big blocks of snow, I got a sudden sharp pain in my right side. I went in the house and sat down until it subsided, then went back to finish the job, however, I did slow down some.

On weekends, Kenneth and I worked together getting ready for the holidays. We baked cookies, and I made Mama's favorite confection-style fruit cake in time to send for Christmas. I packaged everything ready to take to the post office and mail to my family. Then it was time to prepare Christmas for the boys. Kenneth loved this part. Everything he got he anticipated the boys' reaction when they opened it. He found a little bow and arrow set with rubber suction cups on the arrows that would stick to a target board that came with it. This was going to be good. He could teach them how to aim it at the target.

Christmas morning came and I don't know who was the most excited, Kenneth or the boys. After they emptied their socks, they opened what was under the tree. When they opened the bow and arrow set, Michael was especially excited. After Robin found out how it was used, he wanted to get in on the fun too.

While they were learning to use their bow and arrow gift, I went to the kitchen to start breakfast and Kenneth set up the target in the living room. I heard them getting all excited when an arrow actually hit the board. I was looking out the window next to the stove and I could see their reflection behind me. All of a sudden a hole appeared in the window. It was very round and about the size of the little suction cup on the end of he arrow. I turned around and the room was empty, not a soul in sight. Nothing moved. Then a small blond head appeared from behind the big chair.

"Daddy did it," Michael said. All three of them came creeping out from behind the chair. Daddy had to replace a window the next day. It seems the glass was old and "punky" and the rubber suction cup on the arrow was soft and the window did not crack, but the arrow went through, leaving a small round hole.

New Years came and then January 12th which was Robin's fourth birthday. I invited the neighbors for a birthday supper to celebrate. Robin liked deviled eggs so I made a tray of them to go with the dinner. His cake was a train. I decorated a jelly roll to look like an engine. Each person had a small cake decorated like a box car. A licorice whip track went around the table with a box car at each place. He loved it. I went to get the camera to take a picture, and when I came back half the eggs were missing. Robin was chewing like mad, his little cheeks stuffed, his eyes looking big and innocent. He didn't eat much supper but he enjoyed his birthday celebration.

The winter snows were melting and we were looking forward to spring. Kenneth was doing well at his job and, all in all, things were right with our little corner of the world. Every evening Kenneth would come home with a smile on his face. As he turned off the main highway into our drive, I would be getting supper and he would smile and wave. It was such a good feeling.

One evening he turned into our drive, smiled and waved as usual. I saw a sinister grin spread over his face, and instead of slowing down to stop, he accelerated, then slammed on his brakes. He hit a patch of ice under the surface of the soil and slid with a crash into the house. I saw him coming and with two leaps, I was out the backdoor. The little radio, which was sitting on a shelf beside the door, landed in the middle of the kitchen. The smile was gone from Kenneth's face. He came rushing into the kitchen to see if I was okay.

"Are you all right? I didn't mean to scare you. I was just having a little fun and hit a patch of ice. I'm sorry." He had intended to charge up to the house and slam on his brakes to jolt me a little and that darn patch of ice ruined his intentions, and spoiled his fun. The following day, he hooked a chain to the kitchen just above the foundation, attached the chain to the car, and pulled it back on its foundation. It was off almost two inches. The kitchens on the old farm houses were built on almost as an afterthought and were not firmly attached to the main house, which made them movable to a certain degree. So, although it could not be done by hand, the little kitchen was put back on its foundation.

That fall, I got bored and wanted something to do besides housework. One Monday morning, after Kenneth left for work, I made a batch of yeast cake and took samples to the two lunchrooms and one big restaurant in town. I told them that I was taking orders for anything they would be interested in—cinnamon rolls, butter horns, or jelly-filled rolls. The big restaurant asked me if I made pies. I told them I did.

and the following day, I took a sample to them. Overnight, I became a baker. Every day, I delivered rolls and pies to the three restaurants, and on weekends, I made an extra batch of pies for the big restaurant that was connected to a motel. In the evening, I made my pie crusts, rolled them out and stacked them in my freezer to be ready the following day. Early the next Morning, I baked a few of the crusts to be filled with cream fillings and put together at least a dozen fruit pies and four cream or meringue pies. Kenneth made two deep pie carriers with a locking bar in front to deliver the pies safely.

I continued my baking all winter and into spring. I always tried to use fresh local fruits whenever I could. I bought most of them from a local fruit stand owned by a Dutchman who lived nearby.

The big restaurant asked me to bring extra cherry pies one weekend and I was out of cherries, so I went to the fruit stand, to get more. The owner was out of pie cherries.

"What am I going to do?" I asked. "They want cherry pies and I hate to use canned fruits." He told me to take some of his ox heart cherries, put a little vanilla in them and add a thick meringue on top. He told that me his mother made a pie like that when he was a kid and the family loved it.

I thought that it was worth a try. I took some of the big dark ox hearts home and made a pie as he suggested. When I delivered it to the restaurant, I explained that pie cherries were unavailable so I had made them an extra special cherry pie to try at no charge. They loved them and the pies were so popular that I was afraid I wouldn't be able to get enough ox hearts to please them. They were selling whole pies to the motel guests.

I always used the two top shelves in my pie carriers for the meringue pies because Kenneth had made them deeper than the others. I could get six pies to each carrier. I had a good routine going and the pies and pastries were flying out of my ovens.

One afternoon, I made a delivery and had two lemon meringue pies in the top of each carrier. When I got to my destination, I opened the door and there was lemon meringue everywhere. One of the latches had come loose. I took a look at the mess and made an instant decision to quit. Delivering the pies that had not gone scooting, I told them that this was my last day to bring pies; I was closing my bakery business. That was that. I turned my energies in other directions.

CHAPTER 16

Our Last Move Evergreen

Michael was five years old and approaching school age. Kenneth's work was going well, so we talked about finding a place to settle. We wanted to go back to the New Albany area so the boys could go to school where they knew more of the children. We felt comfortable for the first time in our marriage to take on a big debt like a mortgage. Westinghouse was talking about going on strike, so we felt this would be an opportune time to start looking.

The following week we went to New Albany to ask around. Our friends said they would start looking for a place for us. Two weeks later, Westinghouse went on strike, so Kenneth went looking elsewhere rather than waste time. He got on at Sylvania, outside of Towanda and closer to New Albany. One of our friends, Otis Hibbard, had a vacant house that he said they would rent to us while we were looking for a place to buy. We moved just before the rainy season hit. The house had no running water, which meant another outhouse. It sat on a knoll in back of the house. There was an abandoned apple orchard to the right as you entered the driveway. The house was not in the best shape, but it would do while we were looking for a permanent place. We found out how bad it was when the first rain hit. There were leaks everywhere. I grabbed pots and pans and anything I could find to put under the leaks, then pushed the bed into the middle of the room where it seemed the driest. The boys and I sat in the middle of the bed, playing games and reading until the rain stopped. When Kenneth came home, he tried to patch the roof where he could, but it didn't help much.

I awoke one Monday morning feeling as though something was amiss. I rushed through my laundry and straightened the house, and made sure that I had enough groceries for the week. For some reason there was an unusual urgency about getting things done. Tuesday morning, I awoke feeling miserable. I ached all over and I was sure that I was running a fever. I had red spots all over my body including the soles of my feet. I had the measles! Oh Lord! What next. I took two aspirins then hobbled in and got the boys up, fixed their breakfast and went back to bed. Kenneth didn't know if he should go to work or stay with me. I told him to put a bottle of milk, some bananas and cold cereal on the table by my bed, along with bowls for the boys. I was sure I could make it through the day until he got home. I had no problem with Michael as he was content to play quietly beside the bed. Robin was at just the right age, going on four years old, to be very active.

After breakfast, Kenneth left for work. Robin slipped outside when I wasn't looking, I called for but he didn't answer. I dragged myself out of bed. By this time, my feet were very tender and it was all I could do to hobble. I found Robin in one of the apple trees. He was stuck and couldn't get down. I went over beside him and told him,

"Put your foot on this branch." I guided him down the way he went up. When we got back in the house, I got a rope and tied it to the end of the bed and around his middle. No more surprises.

Kenneth finally came home and took charge where I couldn't. After the boys were in bed, I told him the visiting nurse was to come and check on Michael the following day. He was also to have his feet measured for new shoes.

The next day, when Kenneth got the boys up, he called me and said,

"Dolores, I'm afraid Michael has the measles too. He has red spots all over him." I didn't want to hear that. I told him to bring a pitcher of water and some baby aspirin along with the bananas, milk and cereal. He also made some peanut butter and jelly sandwiches wrapped in wax paper. Before he left he tied Robin to the foot of my bed and put the potty chair in the room and we were set for the day.

That afternoon, the nurse came. I tried to pull myself together as best I could, but my feet were a mess. I had put layers of cotton on them and then put on a pair of Kenneth's socks to make it easier to hobble across the floor when necessary The nurse took care of Michael's needs and left. After a week, we were shaky but once again back to normal.

One of our friends in Evergreen came over one evening and said there was a nice house for sale in Evergreen that we might want to look at. We were excited just to have something come up at last. The next evening when Kenneth came home, we ate a hasty supper and went to take a look. The neighbor, Lester Keeny, had the key and took us to a huge house on a hill next door to his home. We drove up the long driveway flanked with grapes, elderberries and brush. Mixed in were a few apple trees. The house was set on the middle of a three level hill. We got out of the car and looked around. Nothing obstructed our view for miles. A three-story barn that had been converted to raise chickens was up the hill a ways behind the house. I loved the look of the whole area. The neighbor's houses were visible but at such a distance that you would have to phone or go outside and call loudly to get their attention. As we walked down toward the house a feeling of excitement came over me. I wanted to turn a cartwheel but I didn't know how, and besides, I was a mother now and had to maintain my dignity. I told myself, "Stay calm," and walked sedately down the steps, one at a time. We entered the house from the back through the kitchen. The kitchen was small but adequate. From there, we went into the dining room. The ceiling and walls were painted a dark forest green, which made it seem small and somber. I would have to fix that right away. I was already thinking of it as my house. We went through the dining room into the living room. To the right was another room that they called a parlor. I never could figure out the purpose of this room. Perhaps, it was used as a library. Off the living room was the door intended to be the front door but the road had been cut through, cutting off most of the front yard, and there was a five-foot drop to the road below. Four flagstones, about four feet square, created a sidewalk that went across the yard to the edge where the road had been cut through. As I looked around, my excitement kept building. Seven gigantic maple trees surrounded the house and the fall colors made the area glow like all the lights of heaven had suddenly been turned on.

We went back in the house and upstairs to have a look at the bedrooms. When we got to the top of the stairs, I opened a door to my right thinking that it was a closet. It was a bathroom. Hurray! A house with a bathroom in a backward farm community. I was falling in love with this place. There were three bedrooms. One was adequate for a small bedroom. To the right was a large room that would be considered the master bedroom and another room that had been partitioned off to make two long narrow rooms. One of these had receding stairs that went to the attic. We took a look at the attic, which was like a third floor; big and roomy with two nice big dormer windows. Going back downstairs we passed the bathroom; I went in and looked out the window. The roof of the kitchen was just below. Standing tall and straight on the roof was a lightning rod.

There were fourteen acres spread out on both sides of the road. Kenneth asked how much they wanted for it. The answer was $9,000. We could not believe our ears; we must have heard wrong. The man told us it was no good for farming so nobody wanted it because most of the people in the area were farmers. The people who owned the house had inherited it and didn't want to continue paying the property tax, so they were practically giving it away.

The next day, we went to New Albany and took out a loan to purchase the house. Iwas so proud standing there beside my husband and signing the papers that would make us homeowners at last. A week later, we moved for what we thought would be the last time into what would be our home the rest of our years.

1956, homeowners at last. We now had a $9,000 mortgage, the monthly payment would be $50.00 a month to the local bank. We were the proud owners of fourteen acres of land, a house, barn, John Deere tractor and a large freezer. We were "standing' tall," as was the saying back West where I came from. I asked Kenneth if we could paint the dining room right away as it was so dark that it was depressing to me. He was all for it so we painted it white the first month we were there. I loved the place. I wandered from room to room enjoying the views from every window. I dreamed of how I was going to decorate each room. It was fall. All the beautiful maples were wearing their vibrant colors and the house glowed from the sun shining through the leaves. Then the leaves came cascading down in great abundance. We raked them in piles and the boys had hours of fun until the leaves were finally raked away and the snow fell, bending the trees down to the ground to make a winter hide-a-way for them to play in. They were always rosy-cheeked from the cold and excitement. This was, our house-well-built, tight and cozy. I hung my little white café curtains at the windows then found a round oak table at my favorite junk shop for the dining room. a I got four unfinished oak captain's chairs and stained them to match. The hide-a-bed went in the living room and my little barrel stave churn lamp sat proudly at one end. The old tub bench I had found in the barn in Nicholson became my coffee table.

Winter was in full swing and I got both boys some long winter underwear to keep them warm. One day, Robin came running in the house and dashed upstairs. I thought he was heading for the bathroom. He no sooner got upstairs when he came walking nonchalantly back down. I asked him what he was doing.

"Checkin' the light' ling rod. Daddy said it was gonna rain and lightling"

"Is it working?" I asked.

"Ya," he said "its standin' up straight." Then he headed out to play. As he passed me, he reached down and tugged on his pants leg

"Are you okay, Robin?" I was always concerned when the boys showed signs of discomfort.

"Ya, Mama," he answered, "but these darn pants is walkin' clear up around my hinges." I couldn't help but laugh; he always had a word that would fit. Even if it was the wrong word, you knew what he meant.

Kenneth came home with a dog one evening. I was ecstatic. It was just what we needed to make us a complete family. It looked like a border collie mix and should be a hardy animal and good with the boys. He was about two years old and accustomed to being outdoors. The boys were thrilled. They decided to call him Lassie. We told them that Lassie was a girl's name and maybe we should call him Laddie. They agreed, so Laddie came into our lives. He fit right in, and when Michael started to school in September, Laddie stayed right by Robin's side until Michael came home. When he saw the bus stop at our driveway, he would run down to greet him.

Deer season came and Laddie turned up missing. One of our neighbors came by on Saturday when Kenneth was home and told him that our dog had gotten shot chasing deer. We didn't have the heart to tell the boys. We told them that Laddie went back to his other home. They missed him for a while but we hadn't had him long enough for them to get attached to him. They talked about him and wondered if his new home was a good one. We assured them that it was.

One of our neighbors had a Boxer mix dog that had puppies. They gave one to the boys and they fell in love with him. They named him Cocoa because of his color. He became Robin's constant companion and followed him everywhere.

Michael was now six years old, time for his second corrective surgery. He was to have a muscle transplant. They would take two muscles from the front of his foot and transplanting them to the back of his ankle which would give him some flexibility. He would be able to move his foot up and down to walk more naturally.

The operation was during the holidays between Christmas and New Year's. He would wear a cast and be in a wheelchair for a short time. We decided to have him tutored for the remainder of the year. His first grade teacher, Mrs. Taylor, volunteered to do the tutoring after school. We would take him to school as the other children were leaving and she would work with him for an hour. I picked him up after she was through. Kenneth helped him on weekends with his reading and he became the best reader of both boys. Robin had his own special talents, which were anything that kept him in motion. Reading would not be his favorite pastime, but he did like to be read to, which became an evening ritual. One series of books that I read them during this long winter was Kippling's *Just So* stories. Robin's favorite was *"How the Elephant Got It's Trunk."* At least once a week, he would pull it out for me to read. In the beginning of the story, it tells how the elephant's child had an insatiable curiosity which meant he asked ever so many questions.

One evening after I read this book to them, Robin went to his toy box to play while Michael was pursuing his favorite game. I called it "question and answer time"

"Mama, what is the stove made out of?"

"Iron." I told him.

"Where do they get the iron?" And on and on went his questions. Robin looked over from his corner by the toy box.

"Michael has a 'satible 'osity' doesn't he, Mama?" I laughed inwardly at his grasp of that big term. "Yes, Robin, Michael does have a 'satible 'osity."

CHAPTER 17

My Hernia Operation And The Ceiling Falls

During that winter, I did a lot of snow shoveling and the pain in my side which came and went seemed to be creeping up on me. I could no longer ignore it. I decided to have the doctor look me over and called to make an appointment. It would be two weeks before he could see me. I woke up a couple of days later and the pain was so great that I had to crawl to a chair to pull myself up. I couldn't wait two weeks. I had Kenneth take me to the hospital. We called some friends to take care of the boys until Kenneth got back.

When we got to the hospital they found that I had a hernia and needed to have immediate surgery. I had the operation the very next morning. When I came out of the operating room, I was put in a room with another woman. For the next few days, I was miserable and missed my family terribly. I became depressed and couldn't eat. A doctor whom I had never seen before came in and talked to me. He said that quite often, after a procedure like this, people felt down and he wanted to know if there was anything they could do to make me feel better. I told him that I just wanted to go home to my husband and children, that I really needed them. He called Kenneth to come and spend some time with me. When he arrived he said the boys were waiting with anticipation for me to come home and they were making a surprise.

I began to focus on the boys and what they had conjured up to surprise me. I tried to picture them at whatever it was they were doing. It perked me up and I finally got my appetite back. I was there a couple more days and the doctor released me. I was pretty sore when I got home. Kenneth fixed a bed in the living room so I wouldn't have to climb the stairs until the doctor gave me the go-ahead.

The boys could hardly wait to show me the surprise. They had me cover my eyes and led me in the living. On the wall was a huge Get-Well card made from scraps of construction paper. I knew by looking at it that it was Robin's idea but Michael had help with the gluing. I loved my boys so much that I nearly burst with joy. I hugged them both and told them how great it was. Kenneth fixed a bed downstairs where I slept until I healed enough to make the stairs.

It didn‘t take long to get my strength back. The doctor told me not to lift anything for a while. The boys became my willing helpers.

That winter, we got a small television. The boys loved to watch, Mickey Mouse, and came running when it was on. Michael sat like a wooden Indian through the whole show but Robin bounced all over the place. I worried about what was going to happen when he started school. I thought, "I'll have to wait and see. Maybe he'd settle down in another year."

One evening after the boys had gone to bed, I went downstairs to watch a little television and relax before I straightened up the house for the next day. I don't remember what I was watching, but all of a sudden a very large patch of plaster, about three feet in Diameter, fell from the corner of the ceiling. It just missed me but covered the television with plaster and dust. I jumped up and backed up as fast as I could. I didn't know what to expect, maybe the whole ceiling was getting ready to drop. I waited a few minutes. When no more fell I grabbed a broom. I realized that I needed something stronger, so I ran to the barn and got a shovel and the wheelbarrow. I started scooping and hauled out plaster for over an hour and finally got it cleaned up. I took a shower and went to bed exhausted.

Kenneth was working nights and would get home at 2:00 a.m. I heard him come in and ran downstairs to tell him what had happened.

I turned on the light and he just stood there, staring at the hole in the ceiling.

"Well, I guess it's time to start remodeling. Come on, let's go to bed we'll face it in the morning." I had no argument about calling it a night.

When Saturday arrived, we were ready. Kenneth backed the trailer up to the porch. taking a square shovel he started shoveling plaster off the ceiling. We had cleaned off about halfway across the room and stopped to rest. We heard a humming sound coming from the ceiling. Looking at each other. Kenneth said,

"Do you hear that sound? I wonder what it is?" He took the shovel and very carefully touched the ceiling where the sound was coming from. A big chunk of plaster fell to reveal a swarm of bees busily trying to load up and move. We vacated the room as fast as possible.

Kenneth went to the neighbors to ask them if they knew anyone who was knowledgeable about bees. They didn't know anyone around New Albany. Kenneth came home, and after scratching his head until his hair was nicely knotted, he took the vacuum cleaner and started vacuuming bees out of the ceiling. After the bees were gone, the vacuum cleaner was loaded with bees and sticky with honey. He threw it in the trailer along with the plaster and lath: it would never clean a floor again. We had all the plaster and lath off the ceiling and started on the walls. When we were through we had uncovered honeycomb clear across the ceiling of the room and up and down one area on the outside wall from the basement to the roof line. There was enough honey to supply the whole town. I got some sterile jars and started rendering honey. They lined my basement shelves in their sparkling amber glory.

It took several weekends to clean things up and get ready for the next phase of our remodeling. We planned on opening the two living rooms to make one long living room completely across the front of the house. The front door opened into a small yard with a sheer drop to the road below. It was a hazard so, We decided to eliminate it and put the front door on the side of the house. We would put a large fireplace where the front door was, extending it from the basement through the peak of the roof. We hired a local mason to build the fireplace.

When spring came, we were ready, and started our demolition in earnest. Kenneth and the boys worked every weekend. During the week I cleaned up after them, stacking lumber that was to be reused.

We discovered the wiring was in bad condition and would have to be replaced With everything else that needed to be done immediately, we put the wiring off until summer.

We heard that the old hotel in Towanda was being torn down so, the next Saturday, we went to see if there was anything that could be used in our remodeling. Kenneth took one look at the beautiful beams which had been holding up the roof of the hotel for years, and got excited.

"Look, Dolores, picture this. We could refinish those beams and put a dropped beam ceiling clear across the living room. It would be very nice and no bees could invade it. What do you think?" I told him that I loved the idea. We bought the beams and some good wiring along with a few other things that Kenneth thought would be useful. We had them deliver the stuff and stack it in our back yard.

By the end of summer, the fireplace was completed with two big picture windows one on each side. What a view. It was spectacular. The front of the house was sealed up and we would be snug for the winter months.

There were a few more weeks of summer left, so we started on the wiring. Living with no electricity for a while was inconvenient but we would manage. One hot Saturday Kenneth went to the attic to drill holes for the wire. He was having difficulty finding the holes when it came time to put the wire through, so he asked me to hold a flashlight up so the light would shine through the holes and make them easier to find. I did as he asked and got a face full of water from the hose that he had positioned just for the purpose of having a little fun at my expense. I quietly grabbed a bucket and filled it half-full of water. When he came jauntily downstairs he asked,

"How come your all wet?" He no more than got the words out when I let him have it, a half-bucket of water right in the face. The war was on. He grabbed the hose and I had the bucket and we went flying around the house. His hose would only let him go as far as the hose would reach, but all I had to do was dip more water from the spring and stay on the opposite side of the house. After we were both drenched, we collapsed in the front yard laughing and cool. The boys watched in amused amazement at their crazy parents. When we caught our breath a bit, we hosed down the boys. We all ended up cool and happy.

Within a few weeks we had electricity downstairs. We would manage with candles and oil lamps upstairs for a while.

The following weekend, Kenneth was out by his stack of beams looking them over and scratching his head, which he did quite often when he was trying to solve a problem. He carried a large measuring tape around with him, snapping it in and out of its casing. It seemed to help him think. Every now and then, he would measure something with it and write a figure down in the little notepad that he carried in his shirt pocket. He came in the house and said he had to run into town and would be right back. He took the boys with him. Off they went on a father-and-son jaunt. About an hour later, they were back. They had some large dowels approximately two inches in diameter and about five feet long, sticking out of the window of the car.

Kenneth went to the barn and got two sawhorses and sat them in the backyard. The boys were helping as much as four-and-six year olds could. They felt they were an important part of what was going on. Robin was holding the measuring tape and Michael was holding the saw. Kenneth had a pencil clutched between his teeth and a square standing by one of the sawhorses.

They worked all afternoon cutting the big beams into lengths. I couldn't figure out what the dowels were for, but I found out soon enough. Kenneth got a drill and started drilling holes in the beams. He stacked everything up and put a tarp over it. It was almost time for supper. He came in and said, "Our project will have to wait until next Saturday. We don't have time to finish it today." I asked what he was making.

"I'll tell you next week; it's a surprise." During the week, I saw him out by his stack of beams several times with a plane, working on them.

The following Saturday, right after breakfast, he began bringing the beams into the house. He laid them carefully on the living room floor one at a time, arranging them the way they would go on the ceiling. There were holes drilled in them here and there and he aligned them so that the holes came together. He had five short beams going the short way across the living room and two long beams the long way on each end of the short beams. He started hammering short pieces of dowels into the holes and the whole thing became one big unit. He looked at me and smiled,

"Now for the fun part," he said. He went to the barn and got a chain. Hooking it in the center of the ceiling to a large hook that he had screwed into the main beam, he attached it to the beams that he had assembled on the floor. Then he pulled the whole thing up to the ceiling. It fit perfectly. After hammering dowels in the holes he had drilled it was solidly attached.

I was totally amazed at what he had done and it all made sense. How he figured it out, I will never know. It was beautiful and all we had to do was put the sheet rock on the ceiling between the beams. I was proud of my "genius" husband and fixed his favorite supper for him; Sauerbraten, and baked potatoes with baked apples for dessert.

We were making fast progress on the house and decided to put a hold on any more building until after the holidays.

CHAPTER 18

Christmas, Santa and the Dog Sled And The Boys Recital

After Thanksgiving, we took our yearly trek into the surrounding mountains to find the perfect Christmas tree. Saturday, we headed for the hills in the Volkswagen bug. Driving along the country road out of Monroten, we found a nice stand of evergreens. Stopping along the side of the road, we all piled out to start our search.

The boys and I walked off the road and up the hill for a few yards and found a nice stand of trees. One we thought was the perfect tree. I went back to the car and got the saw. Kenneth had gone farther up the road and was still searching. I called to him to let him know that we had found our tree and were cutting it down. He called back that he wasn't through searching yet.

We loaded our tree on the car and, after tying it so it wouldn't fall off, the boys and I climbed in the car and drove slowly along the road looking for Kenneth. He had gone farther up the mountain out of sight. I honked the horn a few times and continued searching for him. We were all looking up the mountain when we passed him standing forlornly beside the road with the most pathetic-looking tree I had ever seen. We stopped and backed up for him. He dropped the tree alongside the road and climbed silently into the car. We drove toward home and after a few miles he said,

"Looks like you got a nice tree." We all agreed it was a nice tree. ***
We had started going to the Evergreen Christian church and they were

planning a Christmas program and wanted to include all the children. Robin was four years old but would turn five in January, so we thought he could handle a part. They gave the two boys a rhyme to learn while ringing a little bell; they were to recite their little piece in unison:

"Ring the bells for Christmas, ring them loud and clear. For this is Jesus' birthday, the best day of the year."

They practiced until they had it perfect, as they ran around the house ringing their bells. I would hear," Ring the bells for Christmas." Kenneth and I knew for sure they were going to be a big hit.

The evening of the program arrived, and they were ready. Dressed in their little suits with the short pants and their shoes so shiny that you could see your reflection in them, we walked into the church.

When the program began, the two of them sat as stiff as the lightning rods on our roof. When it was their turn, they marched boldly up onto the stage, holding their little bells in the air. Kenneth and I were beaming, knowing how perfect this was going to be.

It was silent, every eye and ear tuned to our brilliant sons. Michael started,

"Ring the bells for Christmas," Robin stood silently, ringing his bell with his mouth shut tight, his eyes as big as coat buttons. Michael looked at him, frowned and started over.

"Ring the bells for Christmas." Robin rang his little bell vigorously but no sound came from his sealed lips. Michael stopped, put his hands on his hips, looked angrily at his brother he gave him a jab with his elbow,

"Come on, ya' nut."

The audience went hysterical. They howled with laughter. Our sons had changed the somber Christmas program to one that would go down in church history as the most hilariously funny performance ever.

***

This was the last year that the boys would look forward to Santa Clause. I wanted to make it as believable as possible. I called a neighbor who had several older children and asked her if she knew where I could borrow a Santa Clause outfit. She said they had one and would be glad to lend it. Kenneth had gotten the boys a dog sled for Christmas and I came up with an idea. I would have the neighbors' daughter, Roberta Hite, dress in the Santa Clause outfit and deliver the boys' gifts on the dog sled. Christmas eve there was a full moon reflecting off the new snow. It couldn't be a more perfect night. Roberta had agreed to play the part of Santa with as much Ho! Ho! Ho!-ing as possible. She called when she left her house so I would know to be prepared. I saw her lighted lantern coming in the distance and called the boys. I told them to look out the window and tell me who was coming. They both looked intently out the window. We were all very quiet. We heard "Ho! Ho! Ho!" in the distance and over the hill came Santa Clause pulling a sled loaded with gifts. Two little boys hit the stairs on the run and were in their pajamas and under the covers before she got halfway up the hill.

Christmas was all we had hoped for. A beautiful snow fell for several days. It was perfect weather for the dog sled. I envisioned Robin flying up and down the hills with his dog hitched to the sled and Robin sitting in the seat.

Christmas morning arrived and excitement filled the air. Kenneth and I slept downstairs on Christmas Eve so we would be ready to build a fire in the fireplace early in the morning. We knew from experience that we could not keep the boys in bed for long on the morning of the big day. Kenneth had laid the fire the night before and the boys set a little table near the fireplace with cookies and fresh apple cider for Santa. In the morning, Kenneth woke up and said, in a big loud voice, so the boys could hear him.

"Who ate the cookies?" You could hear their feet hit the floor and much scurrying upstairs.

"It looks like Santa came," Kenneth called up the stairs.

The boys called back, "Daddy, can we come down yet?"

"Wait until I light the fire," Kenneth told them, then he asked,

"Where are the matches?"

"In the kitchen, Daddy" the boys yelled excitedly.

Kenneth had them in his hand but he tromped up and down with his feet to make the boys think he was getting the matches just to add a little suspense to the game. After he had the fire lit, he said, “Okay, the fires going. You can come down now.” Michael wore braces but that didn’t slow him down much; he just sat down and slid down the stairs on his behind. The excitement boiled over with many exclamations:

“Wow!”

“Look at the sled.” Robin rushed over and sat down in the sled,

“Who’s this for, Cocoa?” After the wrapping paper was gathered up and put in the fireplace, and the excitement had died down, the boys ate breakfast and spent the remainder of the day enjoying their gifts.

Kenneth showed Robin how to hook up the dog sled for Cocoa. I watched the goings on out the kitchen window. After the sled was properly attached to the dog, Robin sat in the seat and waited for Cocoa to take him for a ride. Cocoa sat down and waited for Robin to do something, anything would be fine. Robin got up and walked down the hill a ways. Cocoa followed hesitantly, looking at Robin with a puzzled expression. After much coaxing, Robin gave up and came in the kitchen and asked for a hot dog. I gave him one and he put it on a string at the end of a long stick, then held it just in front of Cocoa’s nose and away they went down the hill. When they got to the bottom, Robin unhooked Cocoa and had him sit in the sled as he pulled it up the hill again. A few times was enough for Cocoa, and by the third time they went down the hill, Robin was doing the pulling. After that, Cocoa rode on the sled. The sled was definitely a dog sled. Cocoa owned it. He even slept on it.

CHAPTER 19

Bees
And Our Cow Susie Bell

Winter passed quickly and spring soon arrived. We had been working on the house every minute that we could spare. With spring came the wild flowers. Kenneth got the bright idea to get some bees. The wild plants made delicious honey. When we went shopping one Friday evening, he stopped at the Sears catalog store in Towanda and ordered the bee hives with an instruction book on how to raise them. We would have a constant supply of honey. About a week later, the hives came and he put them together according to the instructions. He painted them white and sat them on the edge of the hillside near the trees. Next, he ordered the package of bees. They came with one queen and the proper number of workers and drones. The book instructed him to put the queen in the hive, then release the other bees and they would join her. Everything went according to plan. The book said to wait until just the right time and he could harvest his honey. When harvest time came, he was to put on light-colored clothing, the netting that went over his head and tied around his neck, and the gauntlet gloves that came up to his elbows with elastic to hold them in place.

While he was getting his gear on, I prepared the cookie sheets to bring the honey-combs home on. To save a little on the cost of the whole operation, we had opted to render the honey rather than buy the expensive electric knife to open the combs. I was ready, newspapers covering each cookie sheet. My pans were on the stove waiting for our first batch of honey.

Kenneth came downstairs wearing a white shirt buttoned up tightly around his neck and his light kaki work pants. He had the screen over his face and a beat up old rain hat on his head. The gauntlet gloves were secured well up over his sleeves above his elbows. He asked where the boys' clips were that they wore around their pants legs when they rode their bicycles. I got them for him and he put them around the cuffs of his pants. After he was totally secure, nothing could get into his hide, not even a gnat. He took the smoker that came with the kit and put some cardboard scraps in it, lit a match to the cardboard and gave it a few pumps of air. It sent up a plume of smoke. He picked up the cookie sheets and set off across the field with the dog at his heels.

I waited patiently for all of five minutes when I heard a yell, a bark and a crash on the porch. I grabbed the door and opened it to see my poor husband now hatless, shirtless, and gloveless. Out in the field was a plume of smoke going toward the heavens. Newspapers were flying with the breeze. The dog was running madly for the barn and safety.

"What happened?" I asked.

"There's a bee inside my shirt." Somehow one bee had gotten inside his shirt. That was the end of the bees. He didn't want anything more to do with them. We harvested that batch and sold the whole set. Some things were not worth the effort.

Shortly after the bees left, Kenneth told me that he was going to get a young Jersey Guernsey heifer, and when she was old enough, he would have her bred and we Would have a nice milk cow. A couple weeks went by, and one Saturday afternoon, a truck pulled into our yard. A farmer whom Kenneth knew, unloaded a young brown heifer. She was a delight, with soft brown eyes. The boys were excited when Kenneth told them she was ours. They immediately wanted to name her. After tossing out all the ordinary names that were used for a cow, they finally settled on Susie Bell. Kenneth made a comfortable place for her in the barn and filled it with sweet new hay for her bed. The boys were in the barn more than they were in the house until it began to get cold. They worried about her being warm enough and Kenneth told them that he would make sure she had enough hay to keep her stall warm. Every day, they took water out for her and brushed her.

One morning, we were eating breakfast when we heard a terrible sound coming from the pasture. Susie Bell was down there with her neck stretched out, bawling like an out-of-tune bugler. Kenneth looked out the window and said,

"I wonder what that's all about!" It went on for about an hour. The phone rang and I picked it up. It was our neighbor wanting to talk to Kenneth. I handed him the phone and he said,

Yes," then paused and said, "Is that what her problem is? Okay, I'll be right over." He turned around and looked at me.

"That was Lester and he wanted to know when I was going to bring Susie Bell to see his bull. I guess she was telling us it's time." He went out and put a rope around her neck. I watched as he led her gently down the road; she was still bawling as they walked along. He was gone for a couple of hours, and when he came back he was leading Susie Bell quietly up the road back to her pasture. Peace had returned to our little acreage.

CHAPTER 20

Michael's Third Operation

Michael turned eight years old on September 25, 1959. He was scheduled to have his third corrective operation in November right after Thanksgiving. This would be on his right foot to release tendons that were drawing his big toe up, making his foot widen so that it was difficult to get a shoe that was wide enough to fit his foot. He would be home in plenty of time for Christmas. On the Monday after Thanksgiving, we took him to the hospital and got him settled in. We talked about Christmas and what he thought Santa would bring this year. He wanted a steam engine or a radio to build. We told him that we'd make sure Santa got the message.

He was to come home about two weeks before Christmas, so we made certain we saved some of the fun of planning things for him. The boys and I always made cookies together and Robin especially liked stringing popcorn and cranberries for the tree.

A week after the operation, Michael was running a slight fever. The doctor couldn't figure it out and said he would have to keep him for another week to find out what was causing the rise in temperature. Michael was worried and asked me if he was going to be able to go home for Christmas. I had to tell him I wasn't sure, but if he had to stay longer we would just wait until he got home to have Christmas. The following day, the doctor opened his cast to reveal a large angry pressure sore on the top of his foot After some aggressive treatment, Michael's temperature came down and he came home the day before Christmas. He was one happy little boy.

We had to let Michael sleep downstairs and that was a big concern for Robin, because he knew that Santa did not come if there were children downstairs. Robin had a plan to fix that. He got a piece of cardboard and a crayon and made a sign for the front door.

"DEAR SANTA. WE HAVE A SICK BOY. I HOPE YOU DON'T MIND. HE'S DOWN STAIRS." He got the hammer and nailed the sign to the front door and went to bed, satisfied that he had done what he could to make sure everything went okay.

All was quiet upstairs when Robin came running down to ask for another piece of cardboard.

"Why do you need another one?" I asked. "You've already put a sign on the door, and Santa will see it."

"But Mama, he might come to the back door." So he put a sign on the back door just to be safe.

Michael had us put a screen up between the couch where he was sleeping and the Christmas tree where Santa would be working. He didn't want his surprise to be spoiled. The following morning, after Robin came plunging downstairs and skidded to a halt on his knees in front of the Christmas tree, ready to tear into things. Michael, sitting in his wheelchair, cried out,

Wait a minute, Robin. Mama and Daddy have to get down on their knees and we have to say a prayer and thank God for letting me come home for Christmas." We all dutifully got down on our knees and said a prayer for Michael's presence with us that Christmas. Kenneth and I wiped tears from our eyes. It was a touching moment. I hadn't realized how worried he was about not making it home in time for the grand celebration.

Michael got his steam engine and Robin got a big Tonka truck plus the other assorted fill-ins that made an exciting Christmas.

Kenneth suddenly remembered something and said,

"Hold it. We're not through here," and dashed out to the barn. I never knew what to expect from him; he was not the sentimental type. He came rushing down the hill from the barn with a new garbage can on his shoulder a big red bow tied on the handle. I had time to compose myself before he hit the door, yelling,

"Surprise!" I smiled and thanked him for being so thoughtful. He knew that we needed a new garbage can and he came through as usual.

For a few days after Christmas, the house was quiet. Except for short trips outside, Cocoa spent most of his time curled up on his sled. Michael was occupied with the steam engine and Robin was moving imaginary things from one side of the room to the other with his truck. Kenneth brought home a stack of plaster board to start finishing the walls and stacked it against the wall in the dining area. Michael had a little corner in the dining room where he had his steam engine set up. While maneuvering his wheelchair into position he bumped the sheet rock and it fell over, smashing his steam engine. Kenneth worked and worked trying to fix it, and did get it to where it would work again, but the stack looked a little out of shape.

When Friday shopping day arrived, the boys carefully put their toys where they would be safe. Since we didn't want to come home to a cold house, Kenneth put extra coal on the fire, so it would be warm when we returned. We were gone for a couple of hours, and when we got back we walked into a warm house. Robin ran in to connect with his truck again. He let out a cry of anguish and came running into the kitchen with his truck in his arms

"Mama, my truck is all ruined." he cried. The wheels were completely melted; they were nothing but strings of plastic, most of it went down the register where he had left it sitting I called Sears and explained the situation and ordered new wheels to be sent. It took about two weeks, but they finally came and Kenneth put them on the truck. All was right again; happy engine noises were echoing through the house once more.

CHAPTER 21

Robin's Sixth Birthday

December was coming to an end the New year was a few days away. Other than Michaels operation the boys had been healthy all winter. Robin would be six years old January 14th 1954 and I had planned a birthday party for him. Because the house was in such a mess from remodeling I decided a hobo party would be fun. I invited about eight of his friends and asked them all to dress like hoboes; they were also asked to each bring a raw vegetable. I gave them a choice of vegetables so we wouldn't end up with all carrots. I cooked a piece of beef for the beginning of a stew they would finish preparing themselves. As each child arrived, I helped them clean and cut up their vegetables and drop them in the simmering pot with the beef that was simmering away on the "camp fire" in the new fireplace. The "hobo" mother had a place to sit by the bubbling pot as a precaution to protect the little hoboes from themselves. Hobo mothers knew how unpredictable small hoboes could be. While the stew was cooking, I had my hoboes spread burlap bags in the middle of the floor in front of the "camp fire." They played games and had a treasure hunt while their stew was cooking. Then I brought out a basket with tin cans, clean and polished, which they were to eat their stew in. Sticks, cut and cleaned from the willow tree, completed their table setting. They sat cross-legged on the floor and ate their stew accompanied by chunks of my homemade "hobo" bread that they pulled off of one big loaf. There was much laughter and clowning around and one little hobo let out a smelly little fart which added authenticity to the camp. Robin's cake was German chocolate baked in a large flat pan, dished up with a spoon and topped with rocky road ice cream. When the party was over Robin gave each one of his guests an apple to put in their bandana handkerchiefs that had been their napkins. These they took home with them. The party was a big success.

Robin began talking about what he was going to do in school and all the things he was going to learn, just as Michael had done. He was going to play baseball and run faster than any kid in the school. I thought to myself, "When Robin starts to school, things will never be the same for that school." He hadn't slowed down one bit. I applied for a job in the school cafeteria to start work when Robin did, so I would be on hand just in case the teacher had problems with him.

February arrived and we were still having some snow but it was not bad. Kenneth was working nights at Westinghouse, and had to travel close to seventy-plus miles both ways. He would leave home at two o'clock in the afternoon and get back around two o'clock in the morning. Winters always made me a little nervous because you never knew when there might be a sudden blizzard.

One night, on his way home, he came around a turn following another car that didn't make it. The young man who was driving was thrown out into the ditch. Kenneth got to him just in time to pull his head up out of the water. He ran to the car and turned his blinkers on, then ran back to see if he could help the injured man. Another driver stopped and Kenneth told him to call for help. He stayed with the young man holding his head out of the ditch, but the poor fellow died before help got there. That bothered Kenneth for a long time. He said, over and over,

"I felt so helpless. There was nothing I could do but hold him." I tried to comfort him by saying;

"What you did was the best you could do, Honey. It was his time to go and he was not alone. That should make you feel good."

"I know," he said, "but I feel so sorry for his family."

CHAPTER 22

Susie Bell Has Her Calf

Winter was finally on its way out and spring was showing its soft muted colors. There were spots of snow here and there and nights were still frosty.

One Saturday morning, Kenneth and I were having our morning coffee and the boys had not come downstairs as yet. We treasured these moments and were relaxed and chatting away. Kenneth got up to get a refill and looked out of the window. Our pregnant Susie Bell had been getting pretty round and we were anticipating the arrival of her calf any day. She was across the road in her pasture. Kenneth took a closer look out of the window and said,

"There's something on the ground down there behind Susie Bell." He looked closer.

"It's her calf. She's had her calf!" He grabbed his coat and was out the door in a flash. I watched him run down to greet Susie Bell and saw her little calf struggling to stand. What a joyful sight., It made a lump come in my throat. I watched as Kenneth rushed to scoop the calf up in his arms. Susie Bell was watching him with a concerned look on her face. He headed for the barn, carrying the calf with Susie bawling at his heels.

"Kenneth," I called out, "let her have her calf. She knows what to do."

"I have a place in the barn for them where they'll be warm and dry," he said and continued on until mother and child were snug and warm in the barn and then she was allowed to take over. For several days Susie Bell nursed her calf. We told the boys that the first milk was for Susie Bell's calf: we would have to wait our turn, and then the milk would look different and we could drink it. Kenneth went to the local feed store and picked out the most expensive stainless steel Bucket that they had. He brought it home and placed it carefully, and with pride, in the middle of the kitchen table. We all stood there admiring it. The next morning, I sterilized the bucket. Kenneth took it and a pan of warm water and soap out to the barn and carefully bathed Susie Bell's udder. With more warm water, he rinsed her thoroughly. I had pans ready as I had seen Mama do at home. I waited patiently for my dear farmer husband to come in with gallons of milk. After a while, I peeked out the window. I didn't see any movement from the barn so I waited some more. Finally, I saw him walking jauntily toward the house. Something was different about him, his shoes were white, not brown as they had been. He came in the house and sat his bucket on the table. I peered in. There was about a half a cup of milk in the bottom and the bucket was covered with white foam. His pants were white from the knees down but he said happily,

Well, that's my first try. I'll get better as time goes on." He gave me his famous smile and I knew that he would get better. Before long, he was bringing in gallons of milk. We couldn't use it all and gave some to the neighbors.

I went to my favorite secondhand store in Towanda and found a Daisy butter churn. My years of making butter for Mama would soon pay off. The boys were fascinated with the process and I had no trouble getting them to help. They both wanted to do the churning and would take turns trying to be the one cranking the handle when the butter finally came. At this point I took over, washed and salted the butter, and put it in small crocks to be stored in the refrigerator. Saturday morning after the breakfast dishes were done, I would put the thick cream in the churn and they would start churning while I started my bread-making. After the first batch of butter was churned, the bread dough would be ready for its 'punch down' then it would go in the pans to be set aside to rise the second time and put in the oven. I always made at least two pizza crusts and a dozen hamburger buns to go in the freezer for later use. Sometimes, in the winter months, I made a big batch of oatmeal raisin cookies to be put In the freezer and doled out for special treats.

When the little calf had been weaned from Susie Bell, Kenneth showed the boys how to feed it from a bucket. They would put their fingers in its mouth until it started sucking. Then they lowered their hands into the bucket of milk, pulled their hands out and the calf would clean up the milk in no time. They loved the task and took turns doing the feeding.

CHAPTER 23

Robin's First Grade
Michael's Second

That summer whizzed by and it was time for school. Robin was getting in gear. I could almost picture a windup key sticking out of his back getting him tighter and tighter as the day approached. I would begin working in the cafeteria on the same day he started school. The first day finally arrived, the bus was to stopped in front of our house. The boys had been waiting for at least twenty minutes. Robin had climbed the tree, built a rock fort, worked his shirt out of his pants and both his shoes were untied. He was ready for school.

When they got on the bus, I could see Robin bouncing around, up and down the aisle. The bus stopped a few yards down the road and the driver went to the back of the bus. I watched him talking to Robin, who then sat down in a seat by the window in the middle of the bus. It proceeded down the road with Robin's head bobbing like one of those wobbly-headed dolls. "Oh boy!" I thought. This is going to be something."

I arrived at school about thirty minutes later. The children had not gone in yet and were still playing outside. I spotted Robin running wildly, being chased by a red-haired freckled-faced kid. Robin's cheeks were red, his hair in disarray and his shirttail flying. The school bell rang and children came plunging in from all directions. My job was to help make lunch for the lot of them, so I got busy with what Mae Waltman, the head cook, had laid out for me. The other helper, Mary

Beardsley, had her assigned jobs and the three of us had lunch ready in time with only one hair in Mrs. Norton's salad. Mrs. Norton was one of the teachers and requested special things for her lunch; we always put her tray in an area where she could pop in the door and it would be ready for her. She would look it over carefully and always find something amiss-a hair or a brown leaf of lettuce so small that it was almost invisible, but she would find it. She would ask for a "fresh tray, please." At 12: o'clock, the children started pouring in for their lunches. The first grade came first with much scuffling and rowdiness. The teacher had her hands full and then some. When Robin came through the line, I hardly recognized him as the little boy who had left the house that morning.

"Hi Mama," he said. Turning to his new little buddy, he said, "That's my mama, She's a good cooker."

The children took their lunches to their rooms to eat, and then went flying outdoors for noon recess. I left after the kitchen was cleaned up, at about 2 o'clock. The boys came home shortly after 3 o'clock. Robin was so wound up that he could barely remain in his chair through supper.

I asked him how his first day at school was. While making shapes out of his bread he told me,

"I have a friend and he's all rusty." This had to be the little red-haired boy with freckles. The teacher was patient and gave Robin a week to try and settle down. She finally resorted to sending him into the cafeteria for short times during school hours to sit under the table, where I could keep my eye on him. Instead of taking as a punishment, He thought it was great and played all kinds of little imaginary games while under there. Robin was Robin; that's all there was to it and he was not going to change. He loved school, however, and the janitor took an interest in him and would take him to the basement and help him build things. He came home with a bird house and proudly hung it in the tree waiting for the birds to build a nest in it. Then came a bird feeder and a couple of small logs with holes drilled in them he stuffed with peanut butter and suet for the birds.

Michael had been tutored for most of his first year, so for him, this was almost like starting for the first time. He was the opposite of Robin, very quiet and placid. His teacher was concerned because he let the other children push him around and he made no attempt to defend himself. One of the boys in his class discovered that, with Michael's braces locked, he was stiff, and if you gave him a shove, he went over like a stick of wood. The teacher called me and asked what I thought she should do about this. I told her to let Michael figure it out. I didn't think he would take the bullying for long and I didn't want to coddle him. He would have to make it in the world on his own some day and I could only advise him.

Michael was a big boy for his age and with the heavy braces, he was pretty solid. One afternoon when I got home, his teacher called me. She was very excited and said,

"I just had to call and let you know what happened this afternoon. When the bell rang for recess, Michael started out the door and Joey tripped him. He went down as usual but he grabbed Joey's pants leg and held on, pulling him down with him. He rolled over and pinned Joey until he promised not to trip him again." It seems that Michael had solved his problem and he became Joey's friend. With this arrangement, nobody dared to pick on Michael. They remained friends all through grade school.

There had not been many handicapped children in this small community and the teachers didn't quite know how to handle certain situations with Michael. Occasionally they would call me to ask how to solve a problem that had come up. The school was a two-story structure with outside stairs that went up to the classroom level. A basement was on the first floor. When they had a fire drill, Michael always wanted to be the first one out and would hold up the whole school while he painstakingly made his way down the stairs ahead of the other children. This worried the teachers and they said if they ever had a fire, the whole student body would be at risk. They didn't know how to solve the problem. I asked them how far down the ground was from his classroom window. They said it was only a few feet. I told them to drop him out the window and the first adult out should go to him and lead him to where they wanted him to go. They tried this solution and it worked fine, no longer a problem.

Work in the cafeteria was a pleasant job. The head cook was a local farmer's wife who went to the same church that we went to. Her name was Mae Waltman. I had gotten acquainted with the other lady, Mary Beardsly, when we lived in New Albany.

The school got lots of surplus government foods to feed the children but they still had to pay for their lunches. Only a few got free lunches and the other children never knew who these few were.

There was a family that lived outside of New Albany that had several children. Their dad had a night job and the mother and father slept late. The children got themselves ready for school. They were always clean but came to school dressed in whatever they could find and always looked like they had just gotten out of bed. One of the younger boys gave the impression that he had made an effort to put himself together. His hair was combed and his shirt tucked in and buttoned. He didn't look as thrown together as his brothers. One morning, before the first recess, his teacher saw him putting cardboard in his shoes. The soles were worn completely through. The following day, she went to Towanda and got him some shoes at the secondhand store. They weren't new but they had good soles. When she gave them to him, he seemed embarrassed but thanked her and wore them all day. When school was out, he carefully put the shoes back in the paper bag that they had come in. He put on the old worn-out shoes to wear home. He refused to wear the "new" ones home. The family was very proud and we suspected that he did not want them to know that he had accepted them.

He always brought his lunch box but never opened it. His teacher got curious and when he went out for recess she looked in his lunch box. She found that it contained one raw potato. He, apparently carried the potato so every one at school would think he had a lunch. The teacher wanted to make sure he had lunch but didn't want to embarrass him. She asked a few students if they would like to help clean up the lunch room. She told them they would have the privilege of having leftover food. She made sure this boy was always selected and told him that he was the best worker they had to do this job. He was always happy to be chosen and made good use of the leftovers.

New Albany was a proud little community and was dedicated to bringing up their children to take pride in themselves and to care for one another. Blue jeans were not allowed for school attire because they were considered work clothes. The boys wore slacks and button-down shirts. The girls wore skirts and blouses or dresses. The children were told that part of their education was learning to be successful and they were to "dress for success" from the first grade on. And as far as I could tell, the children were leaning in the right direction. You got the feeling that there were a few who were not going to make the grade, but not many.

Approximately a mile up the road from our place, there was a family with several children. The father had been injured in a wood cutting accident. They were receiving welfare but the children were very undernourished. I wanted to help them by giving them some of our excess milk, but it was not permitted because it was not pasteurized. I found Out, however, that it was okay for me to give them a glass of milk when they came to play with the boys. They received government surplus foods, such as peanut butter, butter, wheat and rolled oats, brown sugar and molasses, flour, sugar, etc. I talked their mother into letting me make whole wheat muffins with raisins every morning during the school week. They would come by and stand around my kitchen table and eat two or three of those big muffins with peanut butter, along with a tall glass of fresh milk. One cold frosty Saturday morning, the oldest boy came by and wanted to borrow some matches for his father. I told him that I couldn't give him matches and asked him if his father could come and get them. He told me his dad didn't want to go out in the cold. The boy stood there with only a coat on, held closed with a safety pin. He had on a pair of shoes with no laces and no socks. I had a strong urge to give that father a good tongue lashing, but I didn't want to embarrass the boy. I could not understand how a parent could treat his children that way.

Another family living farther up the road had two boys and a girl. Their mother had died of cancer. The father worked in a tallow plant and was away from home during the week. The three children took care of the farm animals and themselves during the week. The girl was around ten years old and the boys weren't much older. The young girl came to church every Sunday; she was very quiet but always neat and clean. She sat up in front of me one Sunday and I noticed that the buttons on the back of her dress did not match and were different sizes but they were sewn nicely in place with black thread. It made my heart ache for her.

CHAPTER 24

Robin Goes Fishing And Builds a Tree House

One of our neighbors had a pond on his property. The boys in the neighborhood liked to go there to fish and they always seemed to catch a few fish. I would see them on Saturday mornings, looking like a string of little gnomes, standing on the bank of the pond with their homemade fishing poles. Their little pointy homemade knit hats pulled down around their cheeks while they patiently waited for a nibble. Robin thought this was great and made himself a fishing pole. One Saturday, I saw him heading for the pond which was right across the road from us. I saw him standing patiently on the bank waiting for a fish to bite. He was there a good hour. The next time I looked he was coming up the driveway with a fish on the end of his pole. He took it to Kenneth and proudly told him that he wanted to have me cook it for supper. Kenneth told him it had to be cleaned first, and if he would bring him a clean board. He would show him how it was done. Robin brought the board and Kenneth had him lay the fish on it. He took out his pocket knife and told him to cut the head off. I was watching from the kitchen window. Robin looked at his daddy with disbelief written all over his face. He looked at the fish and placed the knife on the fish's neck then closing his eyes, with a mighty push, he cut off the head. Opened his eyes he looked at his fish. It had shrunk from four inches to three. Kenneth showed him how to clean and scale it. When the job was done, I had a three-inch fish to fix for supper, counting the tail. We all decided that because it was Robin's first fish, he would get to eat it.

When Robin was home, Cocoa was like his shadow. Where one was there was the other. The summer Robin was eight he asked if he could build a tree house. I thought that was quite a big undertaking for him, but he had it all planned out. I gave him my permission providing all the boards and tools would be stored away by the time school started. He agreed and went to work with all the energy and enthusiasm a little boy could muster. That first summer, his tree house consisted of a ladder up the tree with a board on the first limb to sit on. It grew over the next three summers to a three-walled house with a floor. The last summer, he built a platform on the ground. I wondered what it was for because he already had the house in place. It wasn't long until I found out. He put chains on all four corners of the platform. Next, he sat Cocoa in the middle of the platform and attached the chains to his collar. A chain went up into the tree with a pulley attached. As I watched, Cocoa went majestically skyward up into the tree where he was given a doggy biscuit.

Robin was my daring one and Michael was his protector. constantly pulling him away from or out of trouble. One summer morning, I had cleaned the upstairs and the boys were supposed to be cleaning their room. I started down to get breakfast. When I got to the bottom of the stairs, I looked over to the living room and saw something dangling in front of the window. A pair of sneakers attached to a pair of legs were reaching for the roof of the porch. Robin was trying one of his daring escapes out of the bedroom window. I rushed back upstairs to confront his upper half. When I got there, he was standing in the bedroom in front of the window, looking very innocent. Michael had come to Robins rescue once again. I cautioned, "Boys, if you want to go outside, use the stairs."

Another time, the boys were playing outside. Robin was in his climbing mode and had climbed up on the roof of a little chicken house on the hill beside the house. A small hand plow was sitting at the corner of the building with the plow blades upside down. I heard Michael call,

"Mom, come quick! Robin's going to get hurt." I ran out and there was Robin, hanging by his knees off the edge of the chicken house roof, directly over the plow. If he had fallen, he would have landed head first into the blades. Michael was standing under him with his arms up to catch him. He wouldn't have fared so well either. I ran over and retrieved my son while he was still in one piece.

Michael was not immune to his share of accidents, however. One morning, he came down for breakfast. Standing at the bottom of the stairs, he remarked while looking at a spot on his wrist,

"My teacher said if you get a 'boo boo' and it gets all red and a red line comes from it then you have an infection and you have to go to the doctor and get a shot. I think I have one of them." He looked at me with fear in his eyes.

"Do I have to get a shot?" I looked at his arm and told him that yes he did, and I called the doctor. Michael's fear of shots was the biggest thing in his life. It shot terror through his soul. He began to quake and begged me to do something, anything but take him to the doctor.

"Please Mom." he begged, "can't you just wrap it up?"

"No." I told him the doctor has to take care of it, you have an infection."After Robin was on the bus for school, Michael and I headed for Towanda and the dreaded shot. I told him that the shot would only take a second, and, if he was brave we would go to the dime store and get a model for him to build. I tried to keep his mind on getting the model and thinking about what he would like—an airplane, car, or whatever. He decided he would get a race car and he would paint it red.

When we got to the clinic, the doctor was waiting for Michael with needle in hand. Michael had the shot of penicillin before he even realized it. The doctor looked at his wound and decided to give him a tetanus shot also. That was too much for Michael. He became glued to the underside of the examination table. It took the nurse, the doctor, and me to unglue him. He got the shot and lived to see the model car. Sometimes, bravery comes in very small doses.

CHAPTER 25

Pete the Parakeet

Because it was hard for Michael to get around, I tried to think of things to keep him occupied but not isolated. I went to Towanda one afternoon, and while browsing through Grants Five and Dime I heard the birds in the pet section. I went back to take a look. The parakeets were noisily playing. As I watched them, the sales lady came and asked if she could help me. I explained that I was looking for something to please my son and thought the sassy little birds would be fun for him. She said they were very popular and I asked how they were transported. She told me she clipped their wings so they couldn't fly and sent them home in a ventilated box. I thought about it for a few seconds then she added,

"They come with a book on how to train them." The cages were sold separately. I watched them for a few minutes and then picked out an active little blue parakeet. She clipped its wings and put him in a box. I selected a hanging cage, a bag of seeds and a water dish. With the book on HOW TO TRAIN YOUR PARAKEET, I was all set.

When I got home, I called the boys and told them that I had something they might be interested in. Putting the box on the dining room table when the boys arrived, I opened it and out popped the little parakeet. We put some seeds on the table and watched him for a while. The boys were both thrilled with him and wanted to name him. I suggested we wait a while until he got acquainted with us and then we would pick out an appropriate name for him. I read the book to the boys and they were eager to start training him. We were almost sure that he was a male because he was so inquisitive. According to the book, males were easier to train. We hung his cage in a central location and the boys took him out of the cage often to play with him on the floor. Within a week, he was out of the cage more than he was in, and when the boys came into the room, he became excited. One day, he opened the door of his cage himself and plopped down on the floor to waddle over to Michael, who was sitting on the floor. From then on, he was out of the cage anytime they were home. They named him Pete and he would come when they called his name. He became the most incredible little two-dollar-and-fifty-cent bird we could ever have imagined. In just a few months, he had the run of the house. At night, the boys would tell him that it was time for bed. He would go into his cage himself and they would hang a cloth over it to keep him cozy. In the morning, he would open the cage, hop out and call out, "Pete." Nobody slept after he was up. He demanded attention. On weekends, when Kenneth was home, Pete would have breakfast with him. Kenneth liked dry cereal, especially cornflakes. He would always put a cornflake out for Pete. Pete loved this and looked forward to munching along with Kenneth.

One Saturday morning, Kenneth was late getting up and I heard the whir of little wings come up the stairwell. Then there was the tap-tap-tapping of Pete walking across the hall and into our room. Kenneth was still snoring away when he awoke with a start, grabbing his ear. We heard a sharp demanding "Pete," and the little bird was sitting on the windowsill demanding his morning cornflake. Kenneth dragged himself groggily out of bed and went downstairs to put out one cornflake. Pete was happy and busily devoured his breakfast. Pete had learned one very important lesson: When the need demands it, bite the ear, it brings instant results.

When the boys came home from school, they usually arrived just in time for Mickey Mouse Club on television. There was always a rush to drop their books on top of the freezer in the dining room, and plop down in front of the television, for the duration of the show. Michael was still in braces and his foot stood straight up, making a perfect perch for Pete, who would sit there until the show was over, then the boys would play with him until supper time. One afternoon, they were a few minutes late getting home. They rushed in, as usual, and dropped hurriedly down to watch the show that had already begun. Pete was excited to see them and flew over just as Michael dropped to the floor. His hand came down on the tip of Pete's tail and pulled all of his tail feathers out. Pete looked more like a duck than a bird. He flew to his cage and refused to come out for several days until his feathers grew back. The bird and the boys were more careful after that scare.

Winter came and Cocoa was in the house more. He would come in with the boys when they arrived home from school and lie by the fireplace on his rug. I was concerned about how he would accept Pete. So I thought I should let him know that Pete was an important member of the family. Picking Pete up on my finger, I held him in front of Cocoa, Pete had no fear. He stood on my finger and looked Cocoa straight in the eye. Cocoa looked bewildered and looked at me questioningly.

"This is Pete" I told him, "don't you hurt him." Cocoa looked at the bird and never moved.

"Good dog." I said patting Cocoa."Nice birdie." Pete jumped off my finger, waddled over to Cocoa and stopped right between his paws as much as to say, "You better listen to her." Cocoa did just as he was told. Pete ate with him from his dish and he perched on Cocoa's head to watch television. Pete felt very safe with the dog. When spring arrived, we put in a big garden across the road in front of the house. I had to do a lot of weeding and chose to do this when the boys were in school. By this time, Pete was a regular passenger on my shoulder. One of his favorite pastimes was to go out on the porch where I had a cloths line and sass the starlings until he got them dive bombing, trying to find the source of their tormentor. After Pete got them all stirred up, he came into the house and watched them from the safety of the windowsill.

I went to the garden afternoon to do my weeding, halfway down the hill, Pete landed on my shoulder. He went to the garden with me, and as I pulled weeds, he dragged them off into the corn. We worked like that for about an hour, and then it was time for me to go up and start supper. I called,

"Pete, let's go," He was having a great time with the weeds and chose to ignore me. I started up the hill. When I got to the top of the hill, he was still not coming.

"Pete, I called, I'm going to get the hose." He hated to be sprinkled with the hose and soon, I heard the whir of wings flying past me. He was on the clothesline when I got to the house.

He loved to be with me in the kitchen when the boys weren't home and was always someplace close by. When I washed my hands, I cupped them to make a basin for him to take a bath. He would flop around for several minutes. We had some soup spoons with round bowls, and when I washed them under the running water, he tried to take a bath in one. He looked so funny because the bowl of the spoon was just about as big as his little chest. He had a hard time hanging on to the spoon handle while he tried to accomplish this feat. He was one inquisitive little bird and took over the whole house as his space. We were allowed to enter in, providing we followed his rules. We used to put the paper boy's money on the top of the freezer near Pete's shiny handle. He would not tolerate this. He threw each coin on the floor, one coin at a time, watching them roll as they hit the floor. The paper boy wondered why we did this until we found the culprit and chose another spot for the cash.

Pete was around for many years, going to school for show and tell, shopping with Kenneth and when my neighbor came to visit, I would often get a call after she got home, telling me he had caught up with her and rode home on her shoulder. I would have to go out and call him back. Most times with a threat of sprinkling him with the hose. He was the talk of the town. One holiday, I got canned walnuts for my holiday baking. The nuts came in small cans with shiny bottoms. Pete found a can on its side and discovered his reflection in the shiny bottom. He struck up a friendship with the walnut cans. One afternoon, I was wrapping gifts on the dining room table. I saw a movement on the floor out of the corner of my eye. A walnut can was rolling steadily along on a journey to nowhere. I looked more closely and saw a pointy blue tail sticking out of the opening. Pete had found a new mode of transportation. That Christmas the boys got an electric train and a pioneer fort. After setting them up, they took a small mirror and placed it in one of the box cars on the train. Presto change-o. Pete became a hobo traveling the rails. When they played with the fort, they put the mirror inside the fort and Pete became an invading Indian—what else?

Another year went by with Pete right in the middle of everything. Spring came, followed by a busy summer with the boys growing taller. Michael spent the summer learning to ride a bike with his braces on. He took a fall and we made a trip to the doctor for him when he suffered a mild concussion. Robin scared me half to death when he climbed the sumac tree on the bank near the kitchen side of the house. I looked out to hear a "Hi, Mom" from somewhere in the tree that was swaying back and forth in the summer breeze. Pete took it all in stride pursuing his game of 'Stirring up the Starlings' and hiding in the corn. Fall came and it was back to school. I did my Christmas shopping and made my Christmas cards in time for mailing. Soon it was time for baking. Early In our marriage, Kenneth told me how his mother would bake boxes of cookies before the holidays, some for the family and some for giving to the church and school. Not to be outdone, I baked in earnest. A dozen Stollen wreaths, six for the freezer to be given to friends and six for parties and family. Cookies galore—hedgehogs, gingerbread boys, Berliner krantz, pfeffernusse, springerle lebkuchen to name a few. In the evening the boys and I made popcorn balls to hang on the tree. The Christmas smells were all through the house and Pete had all the nut cans that he wanted to play with. Saturday, I made my weekly batch of bread, then spent time in the kitchen stirring up at least one batch of cookies. One afternoon, I had taken my ingredients out of the cupboard to start my project while Pete was playing with a nut can. I got the spices that I needed and pushed the door of the cupboard shut with my foot. A few minutes later, I saw from the corner of my eye, that it had not shut completely and had swung open, so I pushed it a little harder to close it. I didn't know that Pete had discovered the spice cans inside and had entered to explore. When the door closed, Pete made a dash for freedom. He made it to the entrance at the same time that the door did. He tumbled out on the floor. The door had hit him breaking his neck. He lay there not moving, I scooped him up and he lay in my hand. I put my face close to examine him and he called out weakly, "Pete," and our dear little bird was gone. I cried for him. My wound was so deep that I could hardly bear it. We buried him along with his nut can at the base of the big maple tree where he loved to sit and sass the starlings. I planted primroses over him when spring came and we mourned for the most delightful pet we would ever have.

Several weeks later, we got another little blue parakeet. We spent a lot of time with him and tried o teach him like we had Pete, but he wasn't the same. We finally gave him to our neighbors.

CHAPTER 26

What To Do With the Barn? We Raise Chickens.

After most of the snow was melted that spring, Kenneth picked a Saturday to clean the eaves troughs on the barn. He came downstairs after breakfast wearing his knitted "meatball" hat salvaged from his army days, his heavy work coat and outdoor boots. I thought, "This looks serious." I loved to watch Kenneth work: he was so careful. He went to the barn, and a few minutes later, came out with our big extension ladder. I watched out of the window from the kitchen where I was kneading bread. He stood the ladder by the barn and extended it up to the eaves. The snow was gone where he was working, but there were still patches of frost under the surface, which made it hazardous. My cautious husband placed his ladder firmly in place and gave it a little shake to make sure that it was seated solidly. He started his climb. With one foot on the ladder, he gave it a shake to seat it more firmly. Stepping up with two feet on the ladder he gave it another shake. Squaring his shoulders and with a satisfied look on his face, he bravely took two more steps up and shook it again, the ladder trembled ever so slightly. Kenneth froze in place as the ladder trembled more vigorously. Kenneth stiffened as the ladder became a fast-moving object. With Kenneth hanging on for dear life, it came crashing to the ground. Kenneth's feet slipped off the rung and the next rung hit him hard across the shins. I was sure that he must have broken both legs: I reached for the telephone. If he didn't get up, I would call for help.

Thank goodness he got up, climbed out of the ladder, rubbed his shins vigorously and headed for the house.

He had been so careful and sure of himself. I was so relieved to see him walking that the scene became humorous. I could hardly keep from laughing at the show he had put on. It was like a horror movie, in slow motion. When he came in the door, he was composed. He didn't want me to know how foolish he felt. "What happened?" I asked. He took one look at me and knew that I had seen the whole scenario.

"You saw me, didn't you?" he said. Then we both had a good laugh. Entertainment is where you find it. I put the coffee pot on and we sat while his shins recovered from their beating.

Later that afternoon, he went back to finish cleaning the eaves troughs and our neighbor, Bob Dibble came by. I saw them standing by the barn, talking. They walked Around, looking the building over from one side to the other. I could tell by all the gesturing that the talk was about the use of the barn. After a while, Bob left and Kenneth came in for another cup of coffee. He was excited, "How would you like to go into the chicken business?" he asked. After my experience at Leigh's, I didn't think either of us would ever want to raise chickens, but here he is asking me. "What are you talking about, Kenneth? chickens would be the farthest thing from my mind."

"Let me explain. Bob told me the feed mill is making an offer to anybody willing to take on the project of raising chickens for them. All we have to do is provide the building and they will provide the feed. We will get paid at the end of the nine weeks, according to the amount of weight they gain per amount of feed it takes to raise them."

"Who will take care of them and how many are we talking about?" I asked. My head was filled with questions. Kenneth explained what Bob and he had been talking about when they were looking at the barn. The plan was to take the stairs out of the center of the barn and put them up the back with a door opening to each floor. This would gain needed space for a feed chute in the center. The chute would have openings on each floor to make it convenient to get to the feed without having to carry it up and down the stairs. Kenneth was so excited about the project that I couldn't help going along with it.

The following weekend, Bob came over with his hammer and saw. Kenneth went out, and soon, I began to see a growing pile of lumber beside the barn. Then it began to disappear and became the new stairs going up the back of the barn. Kenneth came in for his coffee break and said that I should come out to see the progress they had made in just one day. I went out with him when he went back to work and climbed the stairs to each individual floor. It was very solid and safe with a handrail to the top landing.

The next weekend, a blower was delivered and set in front of the barn. Then came a big load of shavings. Bob's wife, Shirley, and I would have the honor of spreading the shavings after they blew them up to the top floor. We would spread them on the top floor first, then push them down to the second floor through the opening, where they had taken out the stairs. They would work on the feed chute the following weekend. Shirley and I had the whole week to spread shavings.

Each afternoon, after I got home from the school cafeteria, we would get our grubbies on and be out in the barn. We finished the first floor and were ready to start on the second. Kenneth had put an old door over the opening to keep us from falling through, but there was a space at the end to push the shavings down to the next floor. It was pretty slow going with the shovels we were using. I spotted another door standing in the corner and got the bright idea to use it like a shovel to push the big pile of shavings down. Shirley got on one end and I grabbed the other and we pushed shavings like a snowplow pushes snow. It was great. The job would be done in no time.

We had the extension ladder up to the opening, with the door covering the other end of the hole. We gave a big shove and I stepped on the door over the hole and disappeared from sight. I had forgotten the door had panels in it and they gave way, I caught my foot on the ladder as I sailed head first to the floor below. My hip hit the metal extension on the ladder, as I went down, breaking my fall, but I took a chip out of my hip. My head hit the bottom doorsill and I was knocked out. I ended up wrapped around the door frame upside down, my feet flapping in the air.

Shirley ran out and called to some farmers, who were cutting hay, to come to my aid. After unpeeling me from the door, the men lifted me onto one of the many old doors they found in the barn and hauled me into the house. I was full of barn dirt and my hair was ratty with hay. I asked Shirley; "What happened?" she said, "You fell through the door." The men called for the ambulance that was parked at the only gas station in town. It was also the local mortuary. I heard one of the men say,

"We'll be lucky if they can find someone to drive. Everyone is out cutting hay this time of year." I asked Shirley to get me a wet cloth to wash my face. I had on the worst old clothes I imaginable, because it was such a dirty job. My head had clear enough to be embarrassed about the fact that I was going to be hauled away looking like a hobo.

While they were waiting for the ambulance, Shirley went home and got cleaned up. She at least looked decent. When she came back, I asked her to call someone to get the boys off the bus before they got home. I didn't want them to come home to an empty house with no mama waiting and Kenneth was at work.

The ambulance finally came and they took me to the big training hospital in Sayre about 70 miles from home. After x-raying me they found no broken bones, only a chip out of my hip, and my shoulder was badly bruised. The back of my head was pretty sore where I had hit the door and knocked myself out. I was put in a large ward with several other women, all supposedly bedfast. They gave me something for the pain but, what I really wanted was to go home and to be there when Kenneth got home, he would be shocked, and bewildered to come home to an empty house. The following day Kenneth came and the doctor told him they wanted to keep me a few days to make sure I didn't have a concussion. I was to stay flat on my back in bed. I told Kenneth to be sure and tell the boys I was okay and would be home soon. He kissed me and said;

"Try to stay out of trouble and, for goodness sake, don't fall out of bed. You scare me, some times. I'll tell the boys your alright, just banged up a little, love you, bye-bye." and he was gone.

I got acquainted with some of the women in the ward the following day. One woman was diabetic and she had gone into a diabetic coma. They were teaching her how to recognize when this was happening. She was on a special diet but her husband snuck things in to her that she was not supposed to have.

The second evening, I was there they brought in an elderly lady. The beds were all taken, so they put up a cot for her. Shortly after the nurse left, she called for a bedpan, no one answered her call. Several times during the next hour she called again, each time getting more anxious.

"Please, some one please bring me a bed pan." Still, no one came and she began to cry. I couldn't take it. I got up and got her the bed pan. I told all the ladies in the ward that they had better not tell on me. The nurse finally came and was very irate.

"Who gave her the bed pan!" No one said a word. The next time anyone from our room rang their bell, the nurse was right there.

I went home the day they delivered our first batch of baby chicks. Kenneth let me dump out the first box. They came tumbling out like little animated Easter fluffs, scurrying and tumbled over one another, and pecking at dust particles in the air The brooders were down on the floor that was covered by a bed of nice fresh sawdust. Surrounding each brooder were corrugated cardboard rings. Inside the rings were the water and feed troughs. Little chicks were running helter skelter. There were two brooders to a floor and 500 to each brooder. Four floors made four thousand chicks. They would grow for nine weeks to broiler size and then be ready for market.

I was stiff and sore for a couple of days but got back into the swing of things very soon. Michael came down one morning and said,

"Mom, I think you should get a parachute to wear to the barn just in case you fall again." I swatted him on the behind with a wooded spoon. He laughed and said,

"Only kidding, Mom."

Nine weeks went by fast and our chickens looked good. They were all cockerels and weighed out above average. The pickers came after dark with their crates and caught the chickens as they bedded down for the night. I had sandwiches and coffee for the men to snack on, and of course, not to be outdone by the other women on what we now called "Chicken Row," I had made a couple of pies. I set up a table on the porch so they wouldn't have to traipse through my house and they devoured everything. The next morning, we went out and looked at our empty barn. There were nine chickens that had escaped. Kenneth caught them, and after butchering them they were added to our freezer for future consumption.

The following weekend, we cleaned the barn to get ready for our next batch of chicks. All the leftover feed had to be discarded, the water troughs disinfected and the whole barn sprayed with disinfectant. New shavings were spread on the floors, and the brooders cleaned and dropped down in readiness for our new babies.

The new chicks were brought in and dumped out of their boxes around the brooders. Chicks came tumbling out of the boxes on the run, chasing light rays and each other. Our second batch of chickens were good but not as profitable as the first batch because they were a mixed breed. Nine weeks went by and we repeated the process of catching chickens. We had a dozen chickens for the freezer this time. After we had raised three batches of chickens, Bob decided to cut down one of our trees to make things easier to maneuver around the barn. Kenneth did not want any of our trees disturbed. There must have been an argument about it because he came in one afternoon and told me that Bob would not be in partnership with us anymore after this round of chickens. I felt sad because I liked the arrangement and I liked Bob and Shirley. They were our neighbors and I didn't want any hard feelings between us. After we gathered the chickens, Kenneth shook hands with Bob and said,

"No hard feelings." We remained friends and had many good times together.

When we cleaned the barn this time we decided that it would be profitable to raise some pigs on the discarded feed rather than dump it. Kenneth came home with two squealing piglets. He made a pen for them in the old chicken house on the hill beside the house; he put the discarded feed in barrels to mix with leftover milk and other additives to make good food for them.

We cleaned out the barn, then had a truck load of shavings delivered for round number four. When Mr. Kipp delivered the shavings, he always stood on top of the truck and pushed them down into the hopper. He stood waiting to push them down, when he slipped and fell, landing on the ground on his back. He must have been made out of rubber, because he laid there for about a minute, then got up and slowly climbed back on the truck to finish his job. When Kenneth came in for his coffee, I asked him if Mr. Kipp was okay. He said,

"He's fine. He has fallen so many times I guess he's used to it and knows how to land."

As this batch of chickens grew, so did our piglets. Kenneth made a pen across the road for them so they wouldn't smell up our yard so badly. They grew rapidly on our chicken feed concoction. When they were ready for market, Kenneth asked Lester Kinney for advice on how to capture them to take them to market. Lester told him that it was a fairly simple task. All he had to do was back a pickup to the fence where he wanted them to go out, open the fence, lower the back of the truck, pull out the ramp that went up into the back of the truck and herd the pigs up the ramp. Then he should close the back of the truck and take the pigs on their way. It sounded simple.

Kenneth borrowed Lester's truck and, following procedures, went through the movements, After backing the truck up to the fence and opening it, he lowered the ramp for the pigs to climb in. The pigs were watching everything with great interest. Kenneth opened the side of the pig pen so they could go up the ramp into the truck. After he had maneuvered them into the right position, one pig found an opening out into the pasture and took off running. The other pig, looking a little bewildered, decided to follow. I was looking down on this whole procedure from the house. The pasture was surrounded by an electric fence which Kenneth was well aware of. He stood, scratching his head and looking over the situation, then tried to run them down. Kenneth was never built for running. His feet were so flat that his toes didn't touch the ground. He ran like he had snow shoes on. He finally scratched that idea.

As I watched, he marched toward the barn and climbed onto his John Deere tractor. At full speed' he chased the pigs around and around the pasture. They finally collapsed in a heap and he was able to put a rope on each one. He got two into the truck and secured. He went to lead the last one into the truck, but it got away from him and ran out onto the road. He made one giant leap and wrestled the pig to the ground. I had to leave the window for a minute and I heard him call.

"Turn off the fence!" I looked down at the road. Kenneth was sitting flat on his behind, his legs stretched out in front of him with the pig on his lap, with all four of its feet flying in the air. Kenneth was yelling,

"Turn off the fence!" He was getting zapped by the fence but he was not giving up his hold on the pig. I ran and turned off the fence but I couldn't stop laughing. The scene was so funny. He finally got the pigs loaded and came in for a cup of coffee before delivering them.

Winter had come and the weather was menacing. The chicken inspector came every week to check on the health of the chickens. He told us that our chickens were healthy but he left medication to put in their water to ward of any disease that could come our way. Coccidiosis was one thing they were concerned about. One night, the wind started to blow and the temperature dropped. The wind was blowing through the cracks in the old barn. We were up almost all night trying to keep the chicken's water from freezing. Kenneth finally got the bright idea to drop the brooders down from the ceiling and turning them on low. He opened the windows a crack to let air in and it worked. Everything warmed up inside, but outside the wind was still blowing strong and the snow was piling up in big drifts. We went to bed and slept until almost noon. There was no school the next day because the snowplow couldn't get through, much to the boy's delight, they had a day off from school to play in the snow.

Kenneth went out and turned off the brooders. The wind died down and everything was comfy and cozy in the chicken house. That night, the wind started up again, wild and furious. Kenneth wasted no time. He dropped the brooders, turned them on low and opened the windows a crack. We went to bed and slept soundly. We were exhausted from the previous night's work and were not aware that the wind had died during the night. We woke up the following morning with a start. It was very quiet outside. Kenneth grabbed his pants, shoved his legs into them and pulled them up over his pajamas. Grabbing his boots, he paused long enough to pull them on. Taking the stairs two at a time, he headed for the barn. I followed him out, and when I caught up with him, he was frantically throwing open the chicken house doors and windows. Steam Was rolling out of every opening. I looked inside the first floor and saw a carpet of chickens lying still and silent. I went from floor to floor and found the same thing on all four floors. Out of four thousand, there were about a dozen live chickens, their heads sticking up like cactus on a desert. Eight weeks of effort was wasted, gone with the drop of the wind. Kenneth borrowed Lester's manure spreader and hauled out floor after floor of chickens to the field below the house. He spread them out on the frozen ground. As soon as the earth thawed enough, he plowed them under. That, my friends, was the end of the chicken business. We never raised another chicken.

CHAPTER 27

The Boys Get Their First Bicycle And Go Christmas Shopping For The First Time

Christmas was coming and we decided that it was time the boys got into the spirit of giving. We gave them each a set amount of money to spend. I told them to make a list of people they wanted to give gifts to. They came up with their school teacher, Sunday school teacher, one friend, Mama and Daddy and each other. We went shopping Friday, a week before Christmas. Both boys made a beeline for the only two dime stores in Towanda; Newberry's and Grants. Michael went to one and Robin the other. On our return trip, they were very quiet in the backseat of the car. When we got home, they made a dash for their room. They were very anxious to get to bed. I called and asked,

"Aren't you boys going to wrap your gifts?"

Robin called down, "No Mom, we can do that in the morning."

The following day was Saturday. After breakfast, the boys got paper and wrapped their gifts. They spent the rest of the day upstairs in their room, coming down only for lunch. My mother's instinct told me that something was going on but I kept my nose out of it. After supper, they were back upstairs again. Robin came down in his pajamas and asked me if he could have the cardboard core from the Christmas paper. I gave him one and back upstairs he flew. They were both in bed by eight o'clock. I became curious and thought that I had better investigate. There were excited whisperings coming from their room.

As I climbed the stairs, they got very quiet. I peeked my head in their door and asked "Is everything okay up here? What's going on?" Robin piped up and said, "We got Daddy a Christmas present, do ya wanna a see it?" The cardboard tube that I had given them was stretched like a bridge from one bed to the other. Of course my answer was, "Yes." Robin tipped the tube up and a white mouse tumbled out on the bed. My mouth dropped Oh! My ! Gosh! I couldn't believe it. I stayed calm; I didn't scream, although my insides wanted to. All I could think of was GERMS! Robin was so excited that his eyes were dancing.

"Won't Daddy be surprised?" I thought he would be more like shocked! Robin looked at me with concern. "There's something wrong with its tail I think I need a band aid." I told Robin that I thought his mouse was sick and I didn't know how to fix it. I suggested he give his dad an early Christmas present. I didn't know if it would live until Christmas. They put it back in the box that it came in. I helped them wrap it in Christmas paper and Robin insisted that it have a big red bow on it. They took it downstairs and presented it to Kenneth. He was definitely shocked but he thanked them for such an unusual gift. He said he would get it some feed the following morning.

Sunday morning, he told the boys the mouse was sick and needed to be put out of its misery. After breakfast, they took it outside, still in its box with the big red bow. They placed it carefully on the edge of the hill. Kenneth took his rifle, loaded with scatter shot and sent it to mouse heaven.

Winter passed without any more surprises. With the beginning of spring Kenneth plowed a big spot for a garden. We planted a large crop of vegetables. I would can or freeze all that I could for the next winter.

We thought it was time for the boys to have a bicycle. We weren't sure about Michael but we wanted to give him the opportunity of trying anyway. We decided to get just one bike for them to learn on, and later, we would add another if necessary. Kenneth and the boys went to Towanda and came back with a nice sturdy bicycle. That afternoon Kenneth took them down to the road to start their lessons.

Every Saturday for a few weeks Kenneth was occupied coaching them. Robin got the hang of it right away. Michael was struggling but he was determined. Kenneth told them that he didn't want them riding when one of us was not with them. Because of the bend in the road, an oncoming car would not see them.

One early Saturday morning, Kenneth went out to the barn while I started preparing breakfast. A few minutes later, I heard him urgently calling me. I ran outside as he was coming up over the hill with Michael in his arms He said, "Get the car. Michael is out cold." That old feeling of fear rose up in my throat. I called Robin and we all climbed in the car and headed for the doctor's office. Kenneth told me that when he started up the hill to the barn, he heard the rattle of metal down on the road. When he went to investigate Michael was lying beside the road tangled up in the bike, and he was unconscious. Michael tried to sit up;

"What happened?" he asked, I told him that he fell on his bike and hit his head. He looked bewildered and asked, "Where's my shoe?" We then noticed that his shoe was gone. It must have come off when he fell.

The doctor checked him over and found a cracked cheekbone. He told me to keep him in bed for a day and to put a brick under the foot of his bed to elevate it. If he started throwing up to bring him back because that would be an indication his injury was more serious and they would have to hospitalize him. By the next day, his face was black and blue and his eye was swollen shut but he was back on the bike again. By the end of summer, he had conquered the monster and was riding well.

That summer, the school offered a cooking class each Saturday throughout the summer, conducted by the local power company, Reddy Kilowatt. Michael and his buddy Gary decided that they would join. One afternoon, he came home disgusted. The kids were throwing carrots at each other and Gary and he didn't think that was right. That didn't stop them; however, they loved the parties afterward and eating their creations.

One afternoon, he headed for New Albany for the cooking class. He had been gone about three quarters of an hour when I saw a pickup come into our yard with a bicycle in the back. The door on the passenger's side opened and out popped Michael with a towel over his head. Blood was streaming down his face and he was yelling,

"I'm okay, Mom, just a little cut." I ran out to see what had happened. He told me that he had taken a longer road to the school, one that went down to the main highway. When he was almost there, he came to a sharp turn in the road going downhill. The brush cutter had gone by that morning and cut the brush along the roadside leaving sharp cut ends sticking up. He had lost control and had run off the road into the brush, he fell head first into the sharp ends. He had gone to the house at the foot of the hill for help and the owner brought him home. We headed for the doctor's office in Towanda. and had him stitched up, we returned home. After supper he was back on the bicycle again.

CHAPTER 28

Kenneth's Bonus, The Boy's Summer Campout, And Robin Entertains

While Kenneth worked at Sylvania in Towanda, Pennsylvania, he received his first award. They had a suggestion box on the wall and asked the workers to submit any suggestions they thought would make working conditions better. He had put in a suggestion on how to clean a large pipe that the men had to crawl inside to clean. It was a dangerous job because there was always a chance that someone would see the pipe open and close it, not knowing a man was inside. His suggestion was a way to clean it from the outside and make it safer. He got a bonus and he was elevated to a grade A tool and die level. Of course, that called for a celebration, and the following Sunday after church, we went to a restaurant outside of Dushore. I got myself a new outfit and a new hat for the occasion. Robin, always the observant one, waited until we were seated in the restaurant to form his opinion. He looked at me and wisely said, "I like your hat, Mama, it looks like a flower pot." I sat there feeling like an upside-down plant. I thought that has got to be a compliment coming from my eight-year old son. I looked at him; he was smiling up at me. I smiled back and thanked him.

That summer, the boys got interested in the stand of birch and sumac across the road at the bottom of our pasture. They went to play there almost every afternoon. And, of course, Cocoa was always with them. A small creek wound lazily along the length of the pasture, heading towards our neighbor's pond. When the boys were down there playing their voices echoed up to the house. It was a perfect amphitheater. I sat on the porch and could hear the goings on down below. I didn't want to eavesdrop on my boys but it gave me a perfect opportunity to get better acquainted with their private personalities. One Saturday, they had spent all morning down there busy at something.

Around noon Robin called, "Mama!" I stepped out on the porch and answered him. He said;

"Call Cocoa." I called, "Come, Cocoa, here boy." I waited and Cocoa came charging out of the brush on the run. When he got to the house, he was panting with a doggie smile on his face: he was on a mission for his master. There was a rolled-up piece of birch bark tied to his collar. I chuckled to myself: they're playing Indians again. Just like a true Indian, they sent me an important message on birch bark, what else. I untied the message and carefully unrolled it. In crude lettering. it read, "fix us a sanwich, rap it so Cocoa won't eat it. Give Cocoa a bone." I fixed the sandwiches and wrapped them in foil, tied them to Cocoa's collar and gave him a doggie bone. I called Robin to tell him that my task was completed and he called his dog. Cocoa trotted back across the pasture with his bone in his mouth I knew he wouldn't eat it until Robin said the word, "Now." After a few quiet minutes when I knew they were eating their "sanwiches," the "Indians" got busy again. I could hear the crackling in the brush. I went back in the house to finish my ironing before I had to get supper.

Kenneth had been in and out all afternoon, tending to his chores around the barn. When I was ready to start supper I called the boys to stop what they were doing and come to the house and clean up before they ate. Robin called back "Mama, can we have a weenie roast down here, please?" His "please was stretched out in the most pleading tone he could muster.

"I'll ask Daddy." I called back. I went to the barn and told Kenneth what the boys had been up to all day and they had asked if they could have a weenie roast.

Kenneth grinned.

"You mean we get to be 'Indians' this evening,? Tell them the Chief said okay."

I went back to the house and gathered the makings for a hot dog roast. This would be more sophisticated than the real Indians were used to but we wouldn't mention the ketchup, mustard and potato salad. We would just sit around the campfire and say a lot of "ug's."

When we got to the "Indian camp," we found they had put quite a bit of thought in laying out the area. There was a layer of leaves and small branches under the trees. An old sheet was stretched over a bent willow limb and tacked to the ground to make a tent. One area was cleared and circled with stones where we were told to build the campfire. Big Chief Kenneth got busy and in true Indian fashion, with many ug's along the way laid the wood for the fire. Rubbing two sticks called matches together, he lit the kindling and presto! a true Indian fire was soon blazing away. We had a delightful evening with the boys and after they showed us around the camp, they asked if they could spend the night down there. I knew from my childhood that this was very important to them, and of course we said they could. They each had a flashlight and the night was very warm. I told them there was only one condition. If they decided to come to the house, they must take baths before sleeping in their beds. They agreed to that, but assured us that they would not be up until the sun rose the following morning. We started to leave and Michael said, "Just in case we need help I'll hoot like an owl and you come get us, okay?" We agreed and went back to the house and sat outside in the cool of the evening to chat and enjoy the night sounds.

There was a lot of rustling and quiet conversation going on down at the Indian camp for about an hour. As it got later, the evening fireflies came out, darting around in the darkness. The boys' flashlight beams were crossing and crisscrossing in the trees below. Their voices drifted up to us. We heard Michael say, "I heard a noise."

"It was prob'ly a squirrel," Robin said.

"It sounded like something big" Michael answered.

"Be quiet and go to sleep." There was no sound for a few seconds then Michael said "I think it's a bear," followed by a loud, "Hoot, Hoot," and we could hear branches breaking as something came crashing through the brush. We got to the site in time to retrieve Michael as he burst out of the brush in terror. He was doing pretty well in spite of his braces. He came to the house, took his bath and was asleep in less than no time. Robin was not giving up. We sat on the porch until around eleven o'clock then went to bed. I awoke somewhere between two and two-thirty a.m. and saw a light coming from under the bathroom door. Kenneth was snoring away. I got up and peaked in at Michael. He was sound asleep. I quietly opened the bathroom door and there sat a very disgruntled Robin in the bathtub. He had finally given up, no more camping for that night. When morning came, there was no sound of early morning rustlings from the boys room. I let them sleep until they were ready to come down on their own. They sat, quietly eating breakfast.

"Darn you, Mike, we could have stayed all night but you had to get spooky." Robin said breaking the morning silence.

Michael just sat there, saying nothing. He finally came up with, "Next time we can take our BB guns." I thought to myself, "Oh no you won't!"

Robin came home from school one evening and could hardly wait for supper to be over. He made many trips to the cellar carrying magazines, a cardboard box, drop cord, etcetera. After supper was over, he disappeared into the basement. He had a project going for sure. I cleaned up the supper dishes and went to the living room. Sitting on the couch I settled in for some reading and Michael contented himself with his stamp collection.

Robin was down there for about an hour when I heard him stumbling up the stairs with a lot of clumping and banging. He arrived in the living room with a cardboard box trailing a drop cord. "Mama, can I borrow a sheet?"

I thought, “Oh boy, this is going to be good.” I answered, “Yes, Robin, do you need some help?”

“I need to hang a sheet over the fireplace and turn out the lights.” he said.

I got a sheet from the upstairs closet and helped him hang it from the mantel. He turned out the lights and positioned his box in front of the fireplace, then plugged in the cord with a light attached. A crude but readable sign appeared on the sheet. It read:

THIS IS A COW

We were going to have a movie about cows. As he turned, a roll of pages from the magazines appeared. moving through the box and illuminated by the light behind it. A Holstein appeared with the caption, THIS IS A HOLSTEIN. More cows rolled by followed by their names. We sat with our eyes riveted on the box, watching as JERSEY, GURNSY, ANGUS, LONGHORNS, and on and on until all of the cows in the magazines had been shown, followed by THE END

CHAPTER 29

A Visit to Oregon
The Boy's First Airplane Trip

Kenneth had a vacation coming and we wanted to plan something special. It had been four years since I had seen my parents and we had made a promise to ourselves that we would try to make it home at least every four years. Michael and Robin were nine-and-a-half and eleven. We thought this would be a good age for them to really get to know their grandparents. Kenneth would get only two weeks of vacation, not enough time for us to drive the distance, but if the boys and I flew, we would have an extra week to visit. Kenneth could come by car and we could drive back and stop at a few interesting places along the way. The boys would have an opportunity to do a little real camping.

We made plans to go two weeks before Kenneth's vacation. The boys were excited to think they were going to fly on a real airplane. We left New Albany early in the morning and headed for New York and Idyllwild airport. It would be a long drive, so I packed a picnic to nourish us on our way. We arrived late in the afternoon, in time for the boys to watch the planes taking off and landing while we waited for our flight to be called. When they called our flight, we gave Kenneth a hug and I told him to be careful on his trip out west.

"Maybe we'll see some Indians and cowboys." Robin said. All they knew about the West was what they had seen in the Western movies that Kenneth had taken them to on his father-and-son outings. They thought it was still wild.

While Michael was recuperating from one of his operations, we were talking about Oregon. After relating some of the ways Oregon developed and how wild it really was at one time, Michael decided that when he grew up, he would become a preacher and go to Oregon to preach in the saloons. After thinking it over for a few minutes, he followed with, "I'll get a real tough guy to go with me so he can beat up on the mean guys if they want to fight." We both thought that would be the smart thing to do.

We got to Idyllwild on time, found our seats and settled for our journey "home."

"Fasten your seatbelts" the flight attendant bellowed over the loud speaker. "We're ready for takeoff." I checked to make sure the boys were secured. Both sat rooted to their seats while she went through her speech. They tried on the oxygen mask and looked for the door to evacuate if necessary. They thought the barf bag was funny and went through the act of barfing several times to the amusement of some of the passengers in our immediate vicinity. Michael was clutching the arms of his seat, looking terrified. Robin watched every move outside the window, and was absolutely glowing with excitement.

After we were airborne, the stewardess came by and asked if we were comfortable. Robin's nose was glued to the window and Michael was slumped quietly in his seat, spent from the ordeal of the takeoff. His eyes were still big, however. The flight attendant asked if we would like some peanuts. They were all for that. This was going be a real party. Robin was as fidgety as ever and went up and down the aisle several times. There was an accumulation of big billowy clouds in the sky and Robin remarked, "They look so soft; I wonder if you can jump in them?" I told him that they only looked that way, that they were like thick smoke, and no, you could not jump in them unless you had a parachute on.

Every time the stewardess came by, Robin would ask her questions. "What kept the airplane in the sky?"

"Where did they put our suitcases?"

"How can they tell if we are going the right way?" and on and on. She finally asked him if he would like to go up in the cockpit and talk to the pilot. Oh! Boy! He was all for that. I gave him permission and he was gone for about ten minutes before he was back to tell Michael all about flying an airplane. (this was 1959 pilots could still be a little lax.) I didn't think Robin would ever wind down but we finally arrived in Medford and were met by my folks.

We had a wonderful week with Mama and Daddy. The boys had an opportunity to explored my childhood home.

The weekend before Kenneth came out, Daddy took us to see my sister Barbara in Washington. The boys had their eyes peeled for anything wild and Western to share with their friends back in New Albany. As we drove, I tried to explain what I knew about the country we were traveling through. When we entered Washington, I told them we were going through Indian territory and this was where a lot of Indians lived. It got very quiet in the backseat, which meant that Robin was thinking. All of a sudden he became very animated.

"Look! Look! Mom, there's an Indian over by that hill, I saw his feathers sticking up." Daddy roared with laughter. We passed a few areas that were pretty rough and the boys just knew this was cowboy land for sure. I vowed to get them some books to let them find out for themselves what the West was really like.

We got to Barbara's house and found her gone. Daddy said, "Lets go in and make ourselves at home. She may be just getting groceries. We were not a family that locked doors. There was no need to with close neighbors all around. When Barbara didn't come back, we found towels and had showers. After freshening up, we went to the town of Wenatchee for supper then returned to Barbara's for the night.

Barbara had five children and was always on the go. We should have known that she might be gone but thought it would be fun to surprise her. I left her a note and we started back to Medford the following day. When we arrived, Mama said that Barbara had called and was disappointed that she had missed us. I called her and we had a nice long talk, promising to see her the next time we came out.

Kenneth arrived that weekend and we had a few days to visit before we would have to cram ourselves into our little Volkswagon bug and head for home. Mama wanted to take us to town for some reason; she wouldn't tell us why. When we got to town, she took us to Sears and bought us a nice big tent trailer that opened out into two double beds. The boys were excited. We had a couple of days left before we would start back, so we let the boys try out the tent for the last two nights of our stay That was their first time sleeping out under the stars all night.

Traveling back to Pennsylvania, we stopped at all the campgrounds along the way. After the first two nights, the boys were running out of room for all the souvenirs they were picking up. Kenneth had to explain to them that they would have to make better decisions on what to keep or we would all have to walk and push the car with all the assortment of stuff they were collecting. We all got a laugh out of that but the boys got the message and began gleaning what they had and started gathering smaller items. Michael's interest was in natural items, such as lava, obsidian, pumice stone, petrified wood, mosses, etc. Robin's stash consisted of deer antlers, a bird wing, fungus from a tree, rocks that were pretty in the streams, but when dried, they were just rocks. We stopped at Yellowstone National Park and they saw Old Faithful blow and watched the bubbling colorful Paint Pot. It was a fun-filled week, and one they would remember for a long time.

CHAPTER 30

Cub Scouts

We were back in New Albany all too soon and it was time to get ready for school again. We thought this would be a good year to get the boys into Scouts starting with Cubs, and I would be the den mother for our neighborhood. A week after school started, the boys and I signed up. We went to Towanda and got the proper Scout uniforms and handbooks. After reading all that I, as a den mother had to accomplish, I braced myself for a wild year of connecting with about ten little boys. We had weekly meetings at our house and once-a-month meetings at the fire hall. During the year, the boys and I learned the Cub Scout oath, the proper way to wear the kerchief, and all the formalities of conducting themselves at the meetings. I was amazed at the transformation of ten rowdy little "harem-scarum" boys when they put on those uniforms. They turned into miniature soldiers, stiff and straight with nary a hair out of place, shoulders back and eyes ahead. Even their feet were frozen in their proper unskuffed, brown scout shoes. Their scarves were straight and true. They knew their oath and repeated it with solemn vigor. The meetings were enough to make believers of all the skeptical moms in town. They made maps of the United States, had soap box derbies, climbed trees and ran races, ate tons of cookies and apples. When the meetings were over my house smelled of little boy sweat and gas. They were the most unabashed little farters I ever heard.

When they made their little race cars, they were required to do some whittling. I was nervous about their using knives, so I got them each a potato peeler, the cheap kind, and they did a great job learning to whittle with them.

Each den was to take its turn preparing a meal for the big get-together once a month at the fire hall. Our den chose to make chili. I got out my favorite chili recipe which called for canned beans, not too hot and not too mild. I gave each boy a task. One boy was so klutzy that the boys decided he should read the recipe and remain seated on a stool for the duration of the chili “cook off.” Our chili was a big success and judging from the aroma surrounding the fire hall, every one had more than his fair share. All the boys got their cooking badge to sew on their uniform sashes. The big scout leaders came once a year to check on the boys, making sure they were wearing the proper uniforms and could repeat their oaths. Michael had just had an operation on his foot and the toe of his shoe had to be cut out to allow his foot to heal. When he stood up for inspection, his shoulders were back and his feet placed firmly side by side. The inspector started from top to bottom: hat angle, scarf properly rolled, shirt tucked in, shoes shined. Michael spoke up, “The doctor had to cut the toe out of my Shoe I hope that’s okay.” He got a perfect score.

CHAPTER 31

The School Outing

In May of 1959, the school planed an educational trip to take the children to Philadelphia, Pennsylvania, to see the Liberty Bell and the place where our forefathers had gathered to sign the Declaration of Independence. The school hired a big bus for the occasion. They needed two volunteers as chaperones to help keep everyone in line. I went along as one of the chaperones. The children's mothers were to send something to be shared for their lunches. They were to bring their own snacks.

At four a.m. on the morning of our departure, most of the children were eagerly waiting at the school long before the bus arrived. They carried cardboard boxes and paper bags with their contributions to lunch. Checking them, I found at least five bean casseroles plus hard-boiled eggs and baloney sandwiches. I made sure they were well-packed with ice around them to protect us all from getting food poisoning. Pickles and potato chips would endure.

After the food was safely stored away, the children clambered on the bus. Their faces stiff and shiny from lack of sleep, they chattered away like so many little chipmunks. Most of the boys scurried to the back of the bus, scuffling to get seats by a window. The girls navigated to the front. There was much shoving and giggling as they all found their favorite spots and settled in. The driver asked for everyone to remain seated until our first stop. He started the engine and a hushed silence fell over the bus. I looked back to see a sea of big solemn eyes staring at me over their pillows. I was pretty sure some of them had never been away from home in their lives. The other chaperone and I sat up front, quietly relaxing and enjoying the silence of the moment. The lull of the bus's motor cast a spell over our little charges. Then in the silence, I heard a small pitiful whimper. Looking back, I checked each child huddled with his pillow. I spotted a little girl sitting by herself. She was peering out the window, clutching her pillow and softly crying. I went back and sat down beside her. I asked her if she was all right.

"I'm scared," she said as she looked up.

"Have you ever been on a trip before?"

"No," she cried.

"Do you have a friend on the bus?" I asked.

"Yes," she told me, "but she's way back there," and she pointed to her friend who was sitting two seats back and looked equally terrified. I asked her if she would like to sit with her. She looked up at me with hope flooding her teary eyes.

"Yes." Her tears subsided as I took her back to sit with her friend. After they were seated, I went back to my seat. It wasn't long before the two of them were quietly giggling. Our first stop was for lunch. After unloading the children, we got out the lunch makings and spread them on three picnic tables in the park. Beans, homemade pickles, bags of potato chips (which, I am sure, were a luxury for most of the kids), baloney and egg salad sandwiches, etcetera. The school had provided bottled pop as a special treat.

One of the quieter boys from third grade hit every bean dish on all three tables. He was having a bean "heyday." After a short baseball game, we were all back on the bus for the last leg of our journey. About an hour on our way someone in the back of the bus said, "Joe! For Pete's sake!" Windows began going up in the boy's section. Some of the boys moved away from the culprit, leaving him sitting all alone in his bean aftermath. Looking back, I saw Joe sitting by himself with a very red face. I asked the driver if he could stop at the next appropriate place that had public restrooms. About 15 minutes later, he pulled into a small museum. The boys nearly stampeded to get off the bus. Joe, however remained seated. I waited until the bus was unloaded and went back to him. The smell was strong where he sat. I asked him if he needed help.

"I shit my pants," he said in a muffled voice, too embarrassed to look at me.

"Don't worry," I said. "That's why I'm here. I'll help you." I got a paper bag and told him to go to the restroom and put his soiled clothes in the bag and I would go to the store nearby and get him some new ones. To save him more embarrassment, I had him wait until the other children were on their way back to the bus to go and take care of himself. I went to the nearest store and got what he needed. I also got a small box of laundry soap and some Clorox to wash his clothes and make the atmosphere a little pleasanter: and, I got a bottle of Kayopectate to take care of his stomach problem. I felt so sorry for that little kid: his humiliation would probably follow him through the remainder of his school years.

After getting the children back on the bus, all was quiet again and we soon arrived at our destination. A guide took us to the room where our ancestors had signed the Declaration of Independence. It was a plain rustic room with high wooden stools at each place at a long table. On the table at each setting was a small wooden box. One of the boys asked why the boxes were there. The guide explained that they were for their Bibles. He went on to explain that, before each meeting, the Bible was opened and read aloud. That was the main reason for coming to a new land, so they would have freedom to worship in their own way. All of the children were impressed and they wrote about this when they returned to school.

As a whole the children enjoyed the trip but decided they would never want to live in a place where there were so few trees. New Albany was their world.

CHAPTER 32

Chickens Again

One of our neighbors, a few houses down the road, had an empty barn and decided to put in laying hens. The barn was converted to four floors and white leghorn chicks were brought in. As the chicks matured, the cockerels were weeded out and put in another small chicken house to raise for broilers. The laying hens were left to complete the maturing process. Nest boxes were installed but not soon enough. The chickens were laying anyplace they felt like laying. I told Neal, the foreman, that my folks back in Oregon had some chickens that laid their eggs on the ground and they put glass eggs in the nests to entice the chickens to use the boxes. Neal told this to the owner and they decided to put any eggs they found on the floor in the nests. It worked and the chickens soon learned to use the boxes.

I happened to go by on the day the egg washer was delivered. The two men, Lester Kinney and Neal Allen, were having a time getting it set up. I took their assembly directions and read them aloud to them, step by step and the washer went together fast. After it was in place, the owner asked me if I would be interested in operating it for him. I would have to help gather the eggs twice a day, wash and crate them, and then roll them into the cold storage unit and spray them to keep them moist. It sounded good to me. It was only a brisk walk from home and it would be while the boys were in school. I told him that I would do it but he would have to get someone to fill in on Sundays. He asked Mrs. Hight, a woman who lived nearby if she would be interested in working the Sundays. She agreed and she would also work when the hens were at the height of their laying. So, here I was again, in the chicken business, but I would not be responsible for any caring of the chickens. That suited me fine.

Every morning after the boys were off to school, I walked the quarter of a mile to the chicken house and gathered eggs. I'd grab an egg bucket, and start gathering with both hands, reaching into two nests at the same time, scooping out what eggs were there. If a hen was on the nest, I had to move fast so as not to get pecked. After the first few days, and having encountered a rat or two that had taken up residence in the nests, I got a long stick and nailed a board on the end of it that was just big enough to fit in the nest. If I came across a sleeping rat, I jammed the stick into the nest with the flat board, swiftly doing away with Mr. Rat. I never physically touched one of the critters, but my fear of doing so kept me alert and moving fast. After gathering eggs from the two top floors, I ran each flat through the washer. At the same time, I gently rolled them in the flats, looking for cracked eggs. When I found one I broke it into a quart jar and put it in the cold room to stay cool. These eggs I was permitted to take home for my own use.

I would put a few flats on the belt that carried them through to be washed, then go to the opposite end, where I took them off and stacked them on a flat wagon. I sprayed them with water and rolled the wagon into the cold storage room. I went through the same routine for the two lower floors. That took up the morning then I repeated the process after lunch. The hens began to lay faster and faster and I was running my legs off trying to keep up The foreman finally had to help gather the eggs but the hens only laid faster. He finely gave in and hired Mrs. Hight to help every afternoon. She picked up her little girl from school at around 2 o'clock and brought her along to wait around until the day's work was done. The morning session would be completed and, with Neal's help, the afternoon eggs were gathered and ready to be washed. Mrs. Hight would stand at the opposite end of the washer and load the eggs on the wagon as they came through. Things were going smoothly and fall was on its way, which meant hunting season would soon open. The city hunters would be swarming. You could always tell them from the locals because they would come in overcrowded cars wearing only the finest hunting attire. While rolling down a country road with their heads hanging out the windows, the great hunters would spot a lone woodchuck. Their cars would come to a screeching halt. Even before the dust settled, they would leap out of their cars, guns aimed and start firing It was frightening, because they didn't seem to pay any heed to the direction they were shooting and could care less what was in their path.

One afternoon, we were franticly gathering eggs when a shot rang out. Every hen in the coop went berserk. It sounded like it was right beside the chicken house. I took the stairs two at a time and burst out the door. There, standing beside the chicken house, watching the cloud of white feathers rising from the windows was a great white hunter. Brand new hunter's boots, pants, spiffy jacket and hat with the flaps buttoned neatly up on top. With his little twenty-two rifle hanging limply over his arm, he was looking off across the pasture through his state-of-the art binoculars.

"Hey, mister," I called out, "do you like your eggs scrambled?" He looked around, surprised to see a real live person. "Huh?" was all he could think of to say. I repeated my question and asked him to move on. "We have chickens in here trying to lay eggs."

He looked surprised and said, "Chickens?"

"Yes, don't you see the feathers flying?" I think it was then that he remembered from his school days that chickens lay eggs, and then they are sent to the market where his mommy brings them home in a box. Wait till he gets back to the city and tells his buddies that he saw a real chicken house.

"Sorry," he finally responded and climbed the one step back into his car and left.

We worked on through fall. Every day now, including Sunday, the chickens were like egg machines. Someone said, "Lay" and they laid and kept on laying. It took both of us plus Neal, the foreman, to keep up.

The winter snows began, quietly filtering down through the bare trees, covering the roads and lanes with fine white powder. When I walked home in the evening it was so cold that it squeaked and crunched with every step. I loved it. It was the most peaceful part of the day. As winter became more earnest, we had to shovel a path to the door and my co-worker's little girl became restless. There wasn't much for her to do but, she liked to stand at my end of the washer and watch me inspect and remove the cracked eggs. The chain that carried the eggs down the line to her mother was just inches away from where she stood. I never dreamed anything could happen. Then, one afternoon, it did, in a flash. She suddenly reached out and grabbed the chain, which would carry her little fingers into the gears that kept the chain moving. I saw what was about to happen and yelled for her mother to turn off the motor. At the same time, I grabbed the chain just behind the child's hand to give her a chance to jerk free. My hand being larger than hers gave her the time she needed but my fingers went into the gears at the same time the machine went dead. I was hopelessly caught. My fingers were trapped in the gears. We had a special wrench hanging on a nail just in case something like this might happen. I didn't want to frighten the little girl so I tried to keep my voice controlled. In a loud, demanding voice, I said, "Get the wrench and release the chain." Mrs. Hight took two steps over to where the wrench hung. The nail was empty. The wrench was gone and the foreman had gone across the road to his house. My fingers were in a vise and the pain was crawling up my arm. "Go to the house and get the wrench from Neal and hurry," I demanded. There was no time for patience-those were my fingers turning blue. She was out of there in a flash, and miracle of miracles she was soon back with Neal and the wrench. They released the chain, and I was freed. I ran out to the nearest snow pile and packed my hand in snow. Other than two badly pinched fingers, I was alright and finished the day. I was puzzled however, about the wrench. It had hung on that nail since the day we started. Why would it turn up missing when we needed it? I found out a few days later. It seems that Neal had had a few words with the boss and, out of spite, decided that he would take his tools home and the owner could get his own tools.

Neal had a grown daughter who had Down's Syndrome. She would wander in and out, sometimes standing at the window eating an apple or orange. She didn't contribute anything to the egg business except to aggravate her father. One afternoon, when their grapes were ripening, she came in with some nice plump grapes and laid them down on my shelf where I put the jars of cracked eggs. She stood looking at me as if she wanted me to say something. I looked at her and said, "Are those for me?"

"Yes." She giggled and told me that she had washed them. I replied, "They look good, Wilma, thank you." I ate a few and she was very pleased with herself. She ate her grapes and I was nibbling at mine as I worked. I had to go to the opposite end of the washer to take the eggs off, and when I came back, I reached for a grape and they were gone. Wilma was standing at the window, downing the last few. I said to myself, "Bless her heart she tried." That's good enough for me.

That Friday, I went to Towanda to do my shopping and the boys went with me. I had a small lump in my right arm that I wanted the doctor to look at while I was in town. I thought it could be a harmless cyst but I wanted him to see it anyway. After getting my groceries, I went around the block to the doctor's office and had him examine it. He told me that it was just a cyst but it should come out. I went into his office the following Friday and he removed it. He said there felt as though there was another one just behind it. Sometimes, he said, there can be several in a string, like hot dogs. He told me that if they resurfaced, to come in and he would remove them, but not to worry as they were no threat. That worked fine for me as long as I knew they were harmless and I could go about my business as usual.

It would soon be summer and school would be out. I planned on staying home for the summer and would resume work in the fall when school started again. I had a couple more months to go and I really was looking forward to the break and having time to do things with the boys.

A few weeks later, I could feel the lump coming back but, thought I would wait until school was out before going in to have the doctor take care of it. Two weeks before the end of school, the boys and I went to Towanda to do our Friday shopping. The grocery cart was loaded and we ready to go through the line when I suddenly felt faint. I told Michael to get the groceries in the car and come around the block to the doctor's office and wait for me. I handed him the money to pay for the groceries and I left to walk to the doctor's office. I explained to him what had happened. He advised me to go home and pack a bag. He wanted me in the hospital the next day.

The following morning at breakfast, I told Kenneth. He already knew that I was going to ask the doctor to remove the cysts, but we didn't expect to have to go to the hospital to have it done. I figured that I would be home by Sunday.

I dutifully packed an overnight bag. We told the boys to stay out of mischief and left them some chores to do. Arriving at the hospital a little after noon and I was immediately taken to my room. A nurse came in to take my vitals, gave me a little gown to put on and said she would be back in a short time. I didn't anticipate any problems, so Kenneth waited for me in the waiting room. I was soon put on a gurney and taken to the operating room. The nurse came in and began preparing my shoulder for the removal of the cysts. We chatted while she worked. The doctor came in and she helped him into his operating gown and surgical gloves. They strapped me to the table, making sure my arms were tightly secured and then cranked the table to the proper angle to make it comfortable for the doctor. An anesthesiologist came in to put me to sleep. The doctor waited as the anesthesiologist prepared to place the mask over my nose. The sudden screaming of an ambulance brought everything to a halt. My doctor was paged and he told the nurse to stay with me as he hurried out of the room with the anesthesiologist. The nurse and I were suddenly alone again.

She explained to me that there was an emergency, and because my doctor was the only doctor at the hospital that day, he had to take the call. So, there I was, cranked to a ridiculous angle, strapped tightly to a table and my nose started to run. I asked the nurse for a tissue and to release my hands so I could take care of my nose. Down on a more normal level, I felt less vulnerable and after blowing my nose several times, my eyes began to swell and I began breaking out in large hives the size of my palm. I was breathing like an old worn-out thrashing machine. The nurse rushed out and was back with a hypodermic needle. She gave me a shot and an orderly hustled me back to my room. The nurse told me that I'd had an allergic reaction to something in the operating room and they would have to do the operation in one of the examining rooms. They would not be able to put me out and would have to do a local. This meant that I would be awake during the operation.

My eyes and nose stopped running, the hives began disappearing and my breathing settled into a natural rhythm, so, I guess the shot had done its job. I relaxed and the nurse and I waited for the doctor's return. When he arrived, I was rolled into one of the examining rooms. My shoulder was numbed and the doctor started the task of removing the cysts.

All I could see were his eyes over his mask and the nurse wiping the perspiration from his forehead. I felt nothing and kept telling the doctor that he was doing fine. I don't know if it helped but I figured if I calmly said, "You're doing fine, Doctor." it might help him get through a difficult situation. Anyway, it took my mind off what I was going through and, I hope, eased the doctor's stress just a little.

The ordeal was finally over and I was put back in my little cubicle again. My shoulder was neatly bandaged and I thought I would be out of there soon. No way. The doctor came in with Kenneth, both looking very serious. Kenneth had a worried expression on his face. The doctor sat down beside the bed and explained that he had to take out more tissue surrounding the cysts than he had anticipated because the cysts had spread and had become malignant.

"Why didn't you tell us this could happen, so that we could have had it all taken out the first time?" Kenneth asked.

"Kenneth, what's done is done. Lets just get on with it" I said. He reached over and patted my foot and looked so serious. I knew he was really worried. I thought; I have got to take better care of myself for my family's sake. I was kept overnight and released Sunday afternoon. The operation left a huge crater in my right shoulder, It was no picnic trying to comb my hair and tie my shoes, but with the boy's help I got through the ordeal.

CHAPTER 33

My Allergies And Worlds End Resort

I had a bit of a problem with spring allergies, which the doctor called rose fever because it came on just about the time the roses were in full bloom. I'm sure the roses weren't the only culprits to cause my misery, but the doctor had a whole shelf of different colored pills to get me through until the first good frost.

The first year I had that problem was shortly after we moved to Evergreen on the hill behind New Albany. I got the sniffles every year in August. The first really bad session I had was when Kenneth put in almost a whole field of tomatoes. They were lush and heavy, beautifully formed and begging to be picked. We took a basket and went to the field to gather our bountiful crop. Kenneth took one row and I took the one next to him. We were plucking the beauties off the vines two at a time. My nose started running and I couldn't keep up with it. It was like a river flowing to the sea. I ran out of tissues and we weren't through picking yet, so I asked Kenneth for his undershirt, to stop the downpour. We finally got the tomatoes picked but by this time Kenneth's shirt was wringing wet, and my eyes were red and puffy. I went to the local doctor, whom the town people said was good with allergies. He certainly knew how to keep them in check. He gave me three different kinds of pills with the instructions to take one kind until it was gone, then go to number two. When that was gone, I was to start on number three, and then come back before I ran out so that he could give me more.

The neighbors said they weren't surprised at my allergies, as just about everyone around had the same problem. There was only one place people could go to get relief when the air was so loaded with pollen and that was to a small resort area called World's End a few miles beyond New Albany, tucked away in the beautiful mountains.

The school children were hired every year to pick the pollen-producing weeds in that area and make it almost pollen-free. There was a magnificent waterfall coming down from the springs in the mountain that created a huge natural swimming hole that was widely used, especially by the people from the nearby cities. A vast park had been created around the swimming hole with camp areas for weekend camping.

The boys were both good swimmers, so we found ourselves going to the park almost every weekend for recreation and relief. What a godsend it was! Sundays we would pack a picnic lunch, and as soon as church was out, we'd head for World's End, staying late into the evening. With Michael's polio, we tried to get him to exercise as much as possible and he loved swimming and would swim for hours. Robin swam some but seemed to find more interesting things to do on the beach.

There were always families with children there and it was often hard to tell which children belonged to which family, because they all banded together to challenge each other's swimming skills.

One Sunday afternoon, I was sitting in a lawn chair watching the children play, and I noticed three little boys about six or seven years old across the pool in a deeper area. They were trying to see who could stay underwater the longest. One would go down and the others would watch until he came up, then another would disappear. As I watched, it suddenly dawned on me that the third little boy was not with the other two, but was bobbing up and down alone, and no one was paying any attention to him. I then realized he was in trouble and unable to stay afloat. I leaped in the water and got to him as fast as I could and grabbed him under his arms. He looked at me with unseeing eyes, like staring fish eyes. He was drowning. I screamed as loud as I could for help and a man was there in no time. He put the little boy over his arm and water shot out of his mouth. He got him to shore and worked on him for a few minutes. By the time I got out of the pool, he was okay and his parents were taking him to their campsite. An hour later, he was back in the pool. Nothing more was said about the incident but I had nightmares for years after. I will never forget those sightless staring eyes.

As for the allergies, they plagued me for the whole season. Sometimes, it was so bad that I had to wear a protective mask when I went outside. I really looked forward to the first frost because that brought relief. One year, it was close to the end of the season and the nights were getting very cold. I had run out of medicine, and the following day was Sunday, I decided to chance it and go without my pill.

We went to church as usual, and when we started home, I began having trouble breathing. I felt as though I wasn't getting air into my lungs. I alerted Kenneth and we headed for the doctor's office, which was in his home. By the time we pulled into the parking area, my feet and legs had gone numb and my hands were tingling. I could stand, but my feet felt like blobs of clay as I clumped toward the doctor's office. Kenneth dragged me in and pounded on the door.

"My wife is in trouble! She can't breathe!" he yelled at the inner door. He burst into the doctor's office dragging me like a sack of potatoes. The doctor was sitting behind his desk talking to one of his patients. The patient fled into the waiting room.

The doctor looked at me and said, "You're breathing too fast, slow down." He put a paper bag over my mouth and nose and gave me a shot that calmed me and I began to get my feeling back.

The old doc looked at his array of apothecary jars filled with pills, each one a different color, and asked me which colors he had given to me before. I thought that was a strange way to dispense pills, but I figured he had his method worked out and that was okay as long as I got relief. I pointed them out and he selected a new series for me.

Then he told me that if he gave me the same pills, I could build up a resistance to them and they wouldn't work for me, so this was his way of keeping track. I was all right after that, but I made sure that I always had enough meds to last until the frost had done its duty and put the pollen away for the winter.

CHAPTER 34

More Remodeling And I Take a Ceramic Course

Our remodeling was coming along fine. We had added a Dutch door off the dining room and a small bathroom off the kitchen. Most of the work was done on weekends and on any extended layoffs at the factory, such as strikes or long holiday weekends. We were making slow but steady progress. Trying to keep the atmosphere of the house as authentic as possible for its age was a challenge. It was built in the late 1800s from trees That were cut and hewn from the property. Some of the boards in the sub walls were twelve to sixteen inches wide. We tried to imagine what it must have been like to prepare the lumber from start to finish. The house was well built with only one corner that had to be jacked up to square it properly.

After the beams were put in the living room ceiling, Kenneth started putting the sheet rock up. It was difficult trying to hold the heavy sheets up while nailing them. So he made a tee-shaped prop, consisting of a long stick with a four-foot board nailed to the end. I would position the prop under the sheet of plaster board and hold it up to the ceiling while he put in enough nails to hold it in place. Then I'd let go of the prop and set it aside until he was ready for the next sheet to go up. He had completed the living room and started on the dining room. I was working from a ladder in the far corner holding the prop in place, when the phone rang. Kenneth asked me to get the phone and he would hold the sheet rock while I was gone. I asked him if he would be okay and he said, "Yes, just get the phone." It was on about the sixth ring by this time. I grabbed the phone and answered,

"Hello, Dolores here." My neighbor across the road was on the line. "I knew you were home, I could see your car in the yard."

"Oh! Hi Myrtle," I said. "Nice you called. Yes, we're home. I'm helping Kenneth put the sheet rock on the ceiling. Looks like we might get finished with it this weekend. I'm really looking forward to painting and then we can start the floors."

"Are you going to paint it the same color as the walls?" she asked.

"No I think I'll keep the ceilings white and choose an off-white for the walls." I heard a strange noise from Kenneth. It sounded as though he was choking.

"Hurry up!" he said. I half-turned toward him, he was pinned tightly to the wall. The sheet rock had slipped and had him pinned by his neck.

"Kenneth needs me. I'll call you back." I yelled, and slammed the phone down. I helped him out of his predicament and he climbed down off the ladder, rubbing his neck.

"Who was that?" He asked. I didn't think you'd ever get off the phone."

"That was just Myrtle. Are you all right?"

He looked at me. "I think it's time for a cup of coffee." I suggested we take the phone off the hook the next time we put up sheet rock. "Good idea," he agreed.

After our coffee break we went back and finished the ceiling. We needed to tape the seams and do the texturing before we could paint. That would be another week end.

Mrs. Taylor, the boys first grade teacher, called me a few days later and asked if I would be interested in going to a ceramic class with her. I had never had an opportunity to do ceramics and it sounded interesting. I told her yes: I would love to go. It would be one evening a week in Towanda and it was a beginners' class. Everyone would start on the same level with no previous experience. There were three evenings open and it was my luck that one evening was Saturday and Kenneth would be home to watch the boys.

The following Saturday I picked up Mrs. Taylor and we headed to Towanda and a new adventure. When we arrived at the ceramic shop, about a dozen ladies were seated around a long table. At each place, there were two brushes, a small bowl of water, three jars of paint-yellow, brown and black-a piece of sand paper and a small putty-colored duck.

The teacher showed us how to clean the mold seam off the little duckling and smooth the area with water. Next, she had us paint the ducks bill and feet yellow. She then instructed us to paint the eyes brown with black pupils and a white highlight. It was over before it even got started. I had finished my project while everyone around me were still mixing their paints to the proper consistency.

I sat looking at my duck, then I picked up the tiny brush noticing that the bristles came to a sharp point. I wet it and dipped it in the black paint. Very carefully, I started outlining feathers. The lady sitting next to me said in a whisper, “You’re not supposed to do that.”

I looked at her, whispering back, “Why can’t I? It’s my duck.” She just shrugged and looked at me as much as to say, “Suit yourself.” After I painted the feathers the way I wanted them I painted some detailing on the legs. I thought it looked pretty good. When the teacher collected our ducks, she looked at mine and remarked, “interesting.” She said she would fire them during the week and they would be ready to take home the following Saturday. I could hardly wait for the next class and our next project.

When I got home, I asked Kenneth how his evening had gone; he told me that he had taken the boys to a Western movie and that’s what they planned on doing while I was at the ceramic class each Saturday.

At the ceramic shop, there were shelves of green ware, the term for items before they are fired in the kilns. I was fascinated. The teacher told us to pick anything we wanted to paint and she would guide us. One shelf, that had figurines of dancing couples from different lands. I thought they would be fun to paint, so I chose a Scottish pair and did them in black watch plaid. The teacher liked them and asked me if I would do one set of each for display so the students could see how they looked when completed. I didn't think that I could take the time to do all of them but the challenge was tempting. When she said, "Do them for me and I will I will not charge you for the lessons." I couldn't pass that up, so I painted all twelve sets for her.

She gave me the paints and dancers to take home so I could them paint during the week, and that way I was able to get them to her faster.

Kenneth was so proud of me that he splurged and got a porcelain kiln and sat it up in the basement next to the clothes dryer. He found an old W.P.A. desk and chair at the secondhand store to put next to the kiln, where I could sit and paint my heart out.

The first Christmas after getting the kiln, I painted a complete nativity set for the church. The pieces were so big that I had to do the camels in two parts and glue the heads and necks onto the bodies with a ceramic glue. The figures were twelve inches tall and the camels were eighteen inches tall. I learned from this project how to add gold. After the nativity set, I did several sets of kissing angels and one little angel with two tufts of hair, which made her look like a little devilish angel. I gave it to a friend for her little girl. Following that came a tea set for my mother, but to get it to her unbroken was a challenge. Kenneth helped me to make a slush out of toilet tissue, it was like paper-mache, packing each piece in it and letting it dry. We put it on thick and told her to soak the items in warm water to release them. I guess she had quite a time revealing her treasures but they arrived safely, not even a chip. After Christmas, I decided to do a tile design around our fireplace. Choosing a pattern from Kenneth's grandfather's china, I modified it to go around the opening. I drew the design on tracing paper and transferred it to the tile, doing one half at a time. While that half was in the kiln, I traced out the second half in reverse and painted so it to be ready to put in the kiln on the following day. The gold had to be done at a lower temperature, so I started putting the gold on the first half while waiting for the other. A storm came up and we had a short power outage. When I took the tiles out of the kiln, they were slightly faded. I didn't notice the difference until I had them completed and put them side by side. I had to do another set to match but I eventually got the job done. It took me a week but the final effect was just what I wanted. I framed the faded set to hang.

The attic in the house was almost a full story, light and airy with two big windows. There was a receding ladder that you had to pull down out of the ceiling to climb up, then you could pull it up after you and be completely alone. Kenneth put some shelves and a chair up there so I could use it as a getaway studio. It was wonderful when I needed some quiet time to paint, read or just be alone, especially in the long winter months.

Sometimes on the weekends, after working hard, I'd go up into my little hide-a-way. The boys would come in and I would hear them call, "Mom!" When they got no answer, they'd ask Kenneth,

"Where's Mom?"

"I think she went for a walk. She'll be back soon," he would answer, and that seemed to satisfy them. They never found my hide-a-way. When I came down, I was ready to take my place as "Mom," refreshed and ready to go.

CHAPTER 35

One Bad Winter

Every season in Pennsylvania had its good side and its bad side. Spring brought the new growth of awakening plant life and the end of winter gloom. The downside was the rains and lightning storms.

Following spring came the joy of summer with its fresh happy colors bursting forth. But it also left moisture in the air from the spring rains that, with the surge of summer heat, brought the unbearable humidity. We felt as though we were covered with glue and took showers several times a day, our clothes hanging limp and moldy on the lines.

Then, it was glorious, glorious, autumn-a glowing beautiful lady, enough to make you want to sing. Lurking on the dark side of the beauty was the dreaded pollen and popping allergy pills for relief.

On the heels of autumn came winter, which became my first love and my worst enemy. Beautiful, soft glistening snow, menacing, silent and unpredictable, beginning with sleet storms that turned the trees on the ridges of the distant mountains to beautiful icy lace. She snuck in one little storm after another, until she was settled deep for her long stay. She would lay her snow blankets down gently at first, then, would kick up the winds that would create wild blizzards to paralyze the world around us.

Kenneth had to drive close to seventy miles to and from work. I worried every time he left the house to face the winter's vengeance. This season was, by far, my worst enemy. When winter came, one never knew when a wild snowstorm would blow up, completely covering the landscape. Roads and fences would disappear into a vast colorless expanse, bleak and without mercy. If you didn't have landmarks to show where you were, you could get lost in the night.

Kenneth left for work at two p.m. and came home around two a.m. I was always uneasy in the winter, especially if blizzards were expected. One dismal afternoon after he left for work, I looked at the sky. It was an ominous slate color and seemed to hang low over the hills. It gave me the chills. An eerie feeling went up my spine. I was uneasy but I got busy with my household chores and put my thoughts aside: no use brooding over something I couldn't change.

The boys had gone upstairs to their room to play. It was quiet, so after I finished my work, I put a bucket of coal in the furnace, and grabbed a book and blanket. I curled up on the couch in front of the fireplace to take advantage of the remaining embers from the evening fire. I had an hour or so to read before bedtime.

At nine o'clock, I called the boys and told them it was time for bed. Looking out the window, I saw that it had started to snow. I wasn't surprised: it had been hovering overhead all day. I put a small rug in Cocoa's favorite spot near the fireplace and headed for bed myself.

At the top of the stairs, I stood looking out the window into the darkness. In the light that was cast through the window, the snow was coming down heavily, shimmering like tinsel on a Christmas tree, with white shiny shafts of snowflakes, each with its own unique shape. I watched for a few minutes marveling at what nature could do. It seemed so peaceful and calming. I knew that as long as there was no wind, it wouldn't drift and Kenneth would be okay. His little Volkswagen bug maneuvered easily over the snow. With its solid bottom, it was like a sled. He may be a little late but he should be home shortly after two or two-thirty at the latest.

Putting on Kenneth's army long johns, for extra warmth, I climbed under a pile of quilts and was soon in la-la-land. In my sleep I rolled on my side and reached out. No Kenneth! I was suddenly, wide awake, I threw back the blankets and turned on the light. The clock said four a.m. Oh! Dear God! Where's Kenneth! I looked out the window into a wild blizzard. Oh! Dear God! Help him!

Running downstairs, turning on the lights as I went. I ran to the kitchen window and looked up the hill where his car should be. I couldn't see a thing. The snow had drifted, completely obliterating the view. I knew that he was out there somewhere, lost in the storm.

With my heart thumping, all I could think of was that he would be very cold when he got home. I had not thought for a second that he wouldn't make it, but I knew in my heart that it would be close. I put the coffee pot on, then ran upstairs and turned the hot water on in the tub. As the tub filled, I ran back downstairs and flipped the porch light on. The wind had piled the snow in great drifts at the back of the house but the porch side was almost bare. With the exception of the boys' room, I had all the lights in the house blazing away. Our house stood on our hill like a beacon. The night was dense and black, filled with swirling snow. Taking the stairs two at a time, I rushed back upstairs and turned off the water. A sudden soft thump on the porch sent me running back down. I grabbed the door knob and opened the door. I was filled with relief to see Kenneth standing there staring at me. Oh! Thank God!

His eyebrows were crusted with snow and he was shaking all over. Dragging him inside, I sat him on the nearest chair and poured him a cup of coffee. He was shaking so badly that he couldn't hold it. Coffee went flying all over. I poured another cup and held it while he sipped some of the warming brew. He looked at me, then put his hand on my arm.

"Thank God you turned the lights on," he said. "I was totally lost. I couldn't see a fencepost, house or anything." I got him upstairs and into the tub of warm water. After another cup of coffee, he begin to relax and stopped shaking. He went to bed and slept all the rest of the day and the following night. I told the boys what had happened and that they should let their dad sleep.

The school bus didn't run the next day but our neighbor, Lester Kinney, got the old snow plow out and cleared the roads, much to the boys' disappointment. They were looking forward to a few more days of hibernation.

When Kenneth woke up, he told me that he had left the car parked about two miles down the road by the Evergreen church. He thought that Michael and he could bring it home. Lester had cleared the road by then and he felt there would be no problem. Michael was thirteen years old and had driven the car on our property but never on the roads. However, Kenneth thought he could handle driving it home from the church, so the two of them climbed on the old John Deere and went to retrieve our little Volkswagen bug.

After a while, I saw Kenneth coming down the road on the tractor. Michael was proudly following him, driving the bug. They were soon parked and all was well again. Michael looked as though he had suddenly grown a few inches. I knew he was bursting to tell his friends that he had driven a car all by himself!

CHAPTER 36

The Boys Learn Responsibility

As Michael got older, he felt more and more that he was being pushed out of things because of his bad leg and I could see that he was beginning to resent it. On one scout campout, his scout leader told him to stay in camp while his friends went into the woods to look for firewood. When they came back Michael had cut down a tree just to prove to them that he could do it. Of course, they laughed at him and made him feel more isolated. I was becoming concerned about his teen years and what they would bring to haunt him.

The school bus came right by the house and the boys had plenty of time to get to the road to meet it. Michael, however, was constantly missing it. I would have to take him to school. After about the fourth time this happened, I sat him down in the kitchen and explained to him that the bus was paid for by the parents to take the children to school. I felt that it was his responsibility, as a child growing up to be an adult, to take advantage of the bus and not miss it when it came by. I asked if he agreed with that. At thirteen he acknowledged that I was right. Then I asked him if he thought I would be wrong if I said I could not take him to school anymore if the bus was running. He said,

"No, Mom, you're not wrong."

"All right," I said. "Would I be mean if I told you that if you wanted to get there, you would have to go on the bus or walk?"

He answered that he would not miss the bus anymore, and if he did, he would walk. For two weeks he caught the bus and was very proud of himself. I told him that he was doing great and I knew he could do it. Then it happened. He missed the bus. I didn't say a word. He came in the kitchen with his schoolbooks clutched in his arms, looking pleadingly at me. I paid no attention. He stood there for a minute and finally said,

"Goodbye, Mom."

I waved at him and said, "Goodbye, Mike. Have a good day." He opened the door and trudged down the driveway to the road. Never looking back, he started his long walk to school.

Michael was still wearing a full-length brace on his left leg. As I watched, he kept walking steadily on. I called everybody on his route and told them that Michael was walking to school, and if they saw him go by to please call me. It took him until noon to make the two-and-a-half miles, but he did it on his own. He never missed the bus again.

I found that this was the best strategy with both boys; lay down the rules and have them agree, then carry them out with no more discussion.

As the boys grew older, I felt they could handle a little more responsibility. One Saturday afternoon, I had some shopping to do. I told the boys that I would like them to do some chores for me while I was gone. Michael was given the task of cleaning the kitchen and Robin was to sweep and clean up the cellar. I figured this would take them a good long time. One upstairs and one downstairs would keep the jobs moving along until I got back.

It was the beginning of kite season and kites were on display in all the dime stores in Towanda. I picked out two big ones and planned on surprising the boys with them. When I got home, not a thing had been done. I didn't say a word. Going out to the car, I brought in the two big kites and holding them out in front of me, so the boys could get a good look, I put them in the closet and shut the door with a noticeable finality. I quietly brought in the groceries and told the boys that they were excused to go outside and play. They knew they were in trouble but didn't know how to correct things. After putting the groceries away, I cleaned the kitchen. Then I headed downstairs to clean the cellar. After finishing I went back to the kitchen and started making supper. Michael couldn't stand the suspense any longer. He came into the kitchen and said;

"When you're mad at us, it's just because you want us to be good, isn't it,

Mama?"

"That's right Michael." He looked at me hopefully.

"Okay, Mama, now can we have our kites?" I looked at him and said,

"No, Michael those are my kites, I earned them." I never said another word.

I never had two boys so willing to help me. All week, they looked for things to do for me but they never once asked for the kites. They finally did get the kites, however, because eventually they earned them. I often brought little surprises home for the boys, but not often enough that they expected them. They would come home from school on occasion and I would have the table set as if we were having a party. The boys would ask, "What's going on?" I would tell them that we were having an un-birthday party. I would put a small wrapped gift at each of their places at the table and have a cake with candles on it for them to blow out. I would explain to them that it was my celebration of how helpful they had been. I usually got them a book or something to go with whatever they were collecting. For Michael it could be stamps or coins, and for Robin, craft items, glue, scissors, paper or a small car. They always had a great time for the whole evening with their new treasures.

When Robin was in the second grade, he would sometimes go next door to play with Mickey, Lester Kinney's grandson. One day, he came home and told me that Mickey had a John Deere tractor with a manure spreader and other attachments to play with in his sandbox. He talked about it so much that I knew he was smitten.

One Friday, while the boys were at school, I went to the feed mill and found the whole set of miniature John Deere implements: Tractor, hay baler, and manure spreader. I brought them home and arranged them in his sand pile at the top of the hill. I watched as the bus stopped in front of the house He got off the bus and climbed the steep hill to the house. As he reached the sand pile he usually looked up to see me in the window. I always smiled and waved at him. That afternoon, I saw his blond head come over the rise and he froze looking at the treasures in his sand pile. Dropping his books right on the spot, he never got to the house until I called him in for supper. He filled me in on what manure spreaders can do and his was the real thing. He made a garage from a wooden box that Kenneth gave him to put his treasures in, to keep them out of the weather, and they got all the attention that a little boy could give them.

With both boys, I had these precious moments to tuck away and bring out whenever I felt the need to be close to them. The years were going by and I wanted to cling to every little memory. Looking back now, I can honestly say that these were the happiest years of our lives. They were also the glue that held us close when things got tough. Like all of life, things do change and not when or in ways that you expect them to.

When Michael turned 15, and had just started high school. He rode the bus to Wyalusing and was away from me for the first time in his life. Robin was still in grade school, trying to decide which way he would go. Kenneth and I had brought them up, as the Bible said.

"Bring them up in the way they shall go and when they are old they shall not depart from it." We had both taught Sunday school and never missed taking the boys to church. In fact, this was the way that the whole town of New Albany raised their children. When they passed the law that they could no longer have prayer in school or teach anything from the Bible, the mothers started classes in the church. Every child who was interested could go to these classes, which were held off the school grounds one afternoon a week for an hour There was only one child in the whole school who didn't attend.

CHAPTER 37

Life Takes a Drastic Turn

Our life took a dramatic change almost overnight. It was a Saturday afternoon right after Christmas. Kenneth was doing some work on the house and the boys were upstairs with their new treasures. Outside, the snow was piled high in big fluffy mounds. It was a beautiful, calm, winter day. We had just had our afternoon coffee break and had resumed our activities when the phone rang. The sound vibrated through the house. We didn't get many phone calls, so I became alert as I picked it up and said,

"Hello."

"Hello, Dolores, this is Mama."

I became instantly excited. "Mama, how nice, how are you and Daddy?" There was a decided pause before she answered. "Daddy's fine but I am not so good."

"What's wrong, Mama?"

She came back with her "keep calm in a crisis" attitude and told me that she had incurable cancer and was going to close her children's home.

My mother had a nursing home for severely handicapped children and I knew how much she loved those little ones. This must be very serious for her to come to this conclusion. Stunned, I reached for a chair and sat listening, hoping for what? I did not know. To close her home, I knew, was the last thing she wanted to do and I had never heard my mother give up so easily. This was serious indeed. I was in a daze.

I heard her say, "Dolores, are you there?" I came to and answered,

"Yes, Mama, I'm here. Why did you wait so long to let me know about this?" She said,

"I didn't want to worry you and besides you couldn't do anything about it anyway, it's the way life is, you know." Then I made a statement that would change all of our lives completely.

"Mama," I said, "you have four daughters, and I can't think of one of us who wouldn't help you if you asked. I also know that closing your home is not what you really want to do. If you need help, just ask, please."

She came back with, "Well, you know Janet is in California and can't be much help. She's not settled herself yet, bouncing all over California. She has just started on her third marriage. And Barbara has her hands full in Washington with eight children of her own"

"Have you talked to Phyllis?" I asked. She said that she had talked to her and she was just short of receiving her certificate of completion from the training hospital in Kansas where she had been working for the past several years. She didn't want to interfere with that. This left me standing in the wings. I told her that I would talk to Kenneth and see what we could come up with to help. She said that would be wonderful, and before I could say another word, she hung up. Mama was like that; when there was no more to say, that was the end of the conversation.

With a heavy heart, I told Kenneth what Mama had told me. He put his hammer down and took my hands. "I had the same thing happen to my mother when I was in the service," he told me. "She didn't have cancer, but she was dying and had no one to take care of her. My brother was an officer in the army and my sister had just married a Marine. The army sent me home to care for her. It was a very sad experience to watch her fade away but, you know, I am so glad I was able to do what I did. I have never regretted it. We will have to do what we can."

"I know." was all I could say at the moment. He patted me on the shoulder and said, "Don't worry, we'll work something out." That evening after the boys had gone to bed, he asked me if I wanted to go and be with her for a while and help her through her decision-making and, if necessary, help her find homes for the thirteen little children she was caring for. I was torn between wanting to go and the longing to keep our situation undisturbed. We had struggled for so long, and now we were settled into a normal family life. The boys were approaching a critical point in their development and I didn't want to change a thing at this point, but maybe this was what would lead us to a more meaningful chapter in our lives. Perhaps this is what life been preparing us for; an opportunity to give back to those who had given us so much.

I thought of the struggle that Daddy and Mama had of raising us and trying to keep a roof over our heads. They had made it, and now, it was our time to give back. We were young and we could always pick up the pieces and go on. I felt that we had to give Mama the hope and encouragement she needed.

After the boys were settled for the night, Kenneth and I talked late into the evening and made our decision to do what we could. Kenneth would have to stay in Pennsylvania and I would go to Medford to be with her until Mama no longer needed me, but what to do about the boys was another problem to solve. We finally decided the boys would have to go with me, because with Kenneth working nights, we couldn't leave them alone for that long. The risks were too great.

The following morning, I called Mama and told her that we would be there in about two weeks. The stage was set for a future that we had never planned for and would turn out to be the most important chapter in our Book of Life.

CPSIA information can be obtained at www.ICGtesting.com
Printed in the USA
BVOW031251310512

291424BV00001B/3/P

9 781462 665860